EMERGENCY MEDICINE PEARLS

A PRACTICAL GUIDE FOR THE EFFICIENT RESIDENT

EMERGENCY MEDICINE PEARLS

A PRACTICAL GUIDE FOR THE EFFICIENT RESIDENT

ADAM J. SINGER, MD

Assistant Professor of Emergency Medicine
Department of Emergency Medicine
University Medical Center
Stony Brook, New York

JONATHAN L. BURSTEIN, MD

Assistant Professor of Emergency Medicine
Department of Emergency Medicine
University Medical Center
Stony Brook, New York

FREDERICK M. SCHIAVONE, MD

Residency Director
Assistant Professor of Emergency Medicine
Department of Emergency Medicine
University Medical Center
Stony Brook, New York

 F. A. DAVIS COMPANY • Philadelphia

F. A. Davis Company
1915 Arch Street
Philadelphia, PA 19103

Printed in the United States of America

Last digit indicates print number: 10 9 8 7 6 5 4 3 2 1

Medical Editor: Robert W. Reinhardt
Medical Developmental Editor: Bernice M. Wissler
Production Editor: Marianne Fithian
Cover Designer: Steven R. Morrone

Library of Congress Cataloging-in-Publication Data

Singer, Adam J.
   Emergency medicine pearls: a practical guide for the efficient resident / Adam J. Singer, Jonathan L. Burstein, Frederick M. Schiavone.
      p. cm.
   Includes bibliographical references and index.
   ISBN 0-8036-0123-9 (alk. paper)
   1. Emergency medicine—Handbooks, manuals, etc.
2. Residents (Medicine)—Handbooks, manuals, etc.
I. Burstein, Jonathan L. II. Schiavone, Frederick M.
III. Title.
   [DNLM: 1. Emergency Medicine—methods. 2. Emergencies. WB 105
S617e 1996]
RC86.8.S58 1996
616.02'5—dc20
DNLM/DLC
for Library of Congress   95-39181

As new scientific information becomes available through basic and clinical research, recommended treatments and drug therapies undergo changes. The author(s) and publisher have done everything possible to make this book accurate, up to date, and in accord with accepted standards at the time of publication. The authors, editors, and publisher are not responsible for errors or omissions or for consequences from application of the book, and make no warranty, expressed or implied, in regard to the contents of the book. Any practice described in this book should be applied by the reader in accordance with professional standards of care used in regard to the unique circumstances that may apply in each situation. The reader is advised always to check product information (package inserts) for changes and new information regarding dose and contraindications before administering any drug. Caution is especially urged when using new or infrequently ordered drugs.

Preface

Emergency medicine became a specialty in the early 1970s. Since then, many fine textbooks on emergency medicine have been published. However, much of the information available is not always practical and applicable to specific clinical conditions. Also, it is impossible to read and digest all of this information in a timely manner before one begins working in the emergency department. These texts, while preparing emergency medicine residents for specialty boards, do not help them prepare for the first few months in the emergency department.

We wrote this manual for the junior emergency medicine resident as well as for rotating medical students, interns, and residents in other departments. Using a practical, simple approach, we cover the majority of acute problems encountered in a busy emergency department. We also cover several issues not always well addressed in other texts, such as how to prepare for an incoming patient with a cardiac arrest, what information to obtain from prehospital personnel, what "labs" to order and when, and how to tell a family that their loved one has died.

Emergency Medicine Pearls is very easy to read and may be completed in a few hours, such as on the night before your "tour of duty" in the emergency department. Although some of our recommendations are controversial, we usually have chosen to address commonly encountered problems so that the inexperienced practitioner will at least have some idea of what to do, especially under the sometimes stressful conditions in the emergency department.

We did not intend for this manual to replace information included in more comprehensive textbooks; it may not improve your grades on the in-service exam or the specialty boards. Instead, we offer general guidelines and clinical pearls to help you deal with some of the more common problems early in your career, and thus minimize your already stressful beginning.

Adam J. Singer, MD
Jonathan L. Burstein, MD
Frederick M. Schiavone, MD
Department of Emergency Medicine
Stony Brook, New York

Contents

1

CHAPTER

Welcome to the Emergency Department

The white rabbit put on his spectacles. "Where shall I begin, please your majesty?" he asked. "Begin at the beginning," the King said gravely, "and go on till you come to the end; then stop."
—Lewis Carroll

The emergency department (ED) is a chaotic place. You may feel that you're in Wonderland, and that everyone around you is as mad as a hatter . . . but if you pay attention, patterns will emerge. We hope this book will reveal some of those patterns before you start, thereby making your sojourn through the ED, or your beginning in emergency medicine, a little easier.

Above all, the ED and its staff are dedicated to the patients streaming through every day: the sick, the injured, and those with nowhere else to turn. When they enter the ED, they are first evaluated by the triage nurse (in some departments, this function is performed instead by a clerk, a paramedic, or a physician). Based on the patients' chief complaints and vital signs, they are then divided into those requiring immediate care, those requiring urgent care, and those who can safely wait. The triage nurse will notify the physician-in-charge of any patient requiring immediate attention. Everyone else gets seen in order of urgency and presentation. Usually there is a chart rack or box into which the paperwork is placed to indicate that a patient is ready to be seen by a physician. Your job will most likely be to pick up the next chart in the rack and to go in to see the patient.

For all of these patients, the emergency physician must answer two questions: (1) "Does this patient have a life-threatening condition?"; and (2) "Where should this patient go?" Keep these questions in mind when you see a patient; the person doing triage is not perfect, and patients' conditions may change while they are waiting to be seen. Before you go through the detailed history and physical (H&P), which is the usual routine of other specialties, ask yourself if there is something you *must do now* to resuscitate and stabilize the patient. Sometimes this is obvious: the teenager with a sprained ankle (you have time); the elderly man in cardiac arrest (*you must act*). Sometimes it's trickier: the 70-year-old woman who comes in confused; the motorcyclist thrown 20 feet through the air who is complaining of abdominal pain. When in doubt, *worry*, and ask the supervising physician to sort out who needs immediate intervention. Always look at the patient's vital signs (usually obtained by the triage nurse; if not, get them yourself). Always make sure that all four vital signs are measured (heartbeat, body temperature, respiration, and blood pressure). Marked abnormalities must be explained and addressed in some way. Also, look carefully at the patient as you enter the room; with experience, this initial impression can tell you most of what you need to know.

Let us now assume that the patient is sufficiently stable for you to begin your detailed assessment. Keep in mind that you'll do a concise form of the H&P. The ED H&P is "directed" to the chief complaint and should be short and concise, but inclusive. Certain situations mandate specific detail. In patients with chest pain, a smoking history (as well as other cardiac risk factors) is relevant; in the woman with right upper quadrant (RUQ) abdominal pain, a history of recent gonorrhea may lead you down a particular path (specifically Fitz-Hugh–Curtis syndrome). With experience and training, you will begin to learn the relevant questions and physical findings. The streamlining of your H&P will serve you in other settings as well. Always note what the patient's chief complaint is. It will have to be addressed in your workup and write-up. It is also very important to find out if the real reason the patient is there differs from the written chief complaint. For example, a patient may complain of headache, but the patient's real question is, "Do I have a brain tumor?"; if you do not ascertain this concern and deal with it, the patient will be upset and the workup and disposition will likely be hindered. Sometimes the "true" complaint will come up while you are taking your history; other times you may need to elicit it with such questions as, "What concerns you the most?" or "How do you expect we'll be able to help you best?" Of course, be careful not to ask these in a challenging manner. Also, be sure to address all nurses' notes or prehospital-care notes.

Now that you have completed the H&P, you should have a pretty good idea of what is wrong with the patient. In 80% to 90% of cases, your disposition will be decided based on the H&P. In the remaining cases, the next step is to decide what lab tests or consultations are needed to determine your differential diagnosis. Also, decide what procedures will be necessary to manage the patient's problem. Does a laceration need to be sutured? Do you need to see an electrocardiogram (ECG) to decide what to do next? In most EDs, at this point you will write orders for the interventions, medications, tests, or x-rays you want, and then communicate with the nurses and ancillary staff to get these things done. Some things you will usually need to do yourself (e.g., suturing). Note, though, that the nursing staff and others are valuable assets for the patient's care. Each person usually has specific duties in the care of the patient, and you will find that they will be far more helpful to you if you work closely and cooperatively with them and include them in the treatment plan. If something must get done soon, and you cannot do it yourself, remember to talk (politely) with the nurse who is taking care of the patient about what needs to be done. (You may find that he or she is already doing it.) Pay attention to the nurse's assessment of the patient, usually documented in a nursing note; you will often find valuable information in there that you did not pick up before.

A few tips on labwork: If you do not know what to order, *ask* somebody, such as the attending physician. When in doubt, for an ill patient, remember the "survival kit" of ECG, chest x-ray, and arterial blood gas (ABG)—the information gained will usually reassure you or point you toward a diagnosis. (Be careful, though, not to indiscriminately "shotgun" labs, because this will often complicate rather than simplify the workup.) When drawing blood, draw one of each type of tube, if possible. It may save the patient a restick later if it turns out that other lab tests are necessary. Putting in a heparin lock and drawing the blood through it saves the patient a second stick for intravenous (IV) access. A very helpful rule: *Order labs early.* Sometimes the patient's disposition will depend on lab results, which take several hours to return; the sooner they are sent, the sooner you will be able to make an appropriate disposition for the patient. In many cases, other services also will need to be involved; this is discussed later in this chapter.

Reaching an exact diagnosis in the ED usually is not possible, nor is it expected. The definitive lab results or procedures, such as blood culture results or an exercise test, may not be available. Nevertheless, you should make an effort to assign a working diagnosis to your patient, both to guide your workup and to aid you in making the appropriate disposition or involving the right consultant. You will become skilled in making a diagnosis with very little information. Using pattern recognition is a valuable tool. For example, in an elderly person with carotid bruits (hence, atherosclerotic disease) and abdominal pain, the astute clinician will at least consider the presence of ischemic bowel.

The next step is disposition of the patient. You have only a few options: send the patient home, admit the patient to the hospital floors or intensive care unit (ICU), or observe the patient in the ED for a short time, usually not more than several hours. This decision usually can be made with only a few test results, although in many EDs the "admitting labs" will be sent off if a patient is clearly going to be admitted, as a courtesy to the admitting service. Notice that the decision to admit will rarely hinge on such tests as a complete blood count (CBC) or an amylase level.

At this juncture, other services (e.g., cardiology or surgery) may be involved in the care of the patient, usually in one of three ways:

- The patient is going to be admitted to that service
- The service will be asked to see the patient in follow-up after discharge
- Specific procedures or advice will be obtained from the service to allow discharge of the patient (e.g., plastic surgery to repair a complex facial laceration)

Specific methods for contacting other services will vary from place to place, as will the political complications (no one likes being called by the ED—it means more work!). The ED attending physician will be your best guide through these thickets. In general, when calling other services, be brief, make it clear why you are calling, and have all relevant data in front of you for rapid reference (such as H&P notes, labs, ECGs, or old chart). If a patient has a primary physician, it is appropriate (and almost mandatory), if possible, to let that person know what your plan is. The primary physician may be a useful source of information about the patient as well.

A word must be said about follow-up: it *must be* arranged for all discharged patients. This can be as simple as telling the patient to call his or her own doctor if any problems occur. In general, though, anyone sent home with a potentially serious problem, such as chest pain or abdominal pain, should be given very clear instructions regarding whom to see or call, when to call, and what specific problems to worry about. For example, a patient with right lower quadrant (RLQ) pain, who seems well enough to go home but might conceivably have appendicitis, could be told: "If the pain becomes more severe or you develop repeated vomiting or fever, come back here immediately. Otherwise, see the surgeon Dr. Jones at 10 AM 3 days from now." Whenever possible, contact the physician you want the patient to see in follow-up, to ensure that these instructions can be carried out in a timely manner. Some EDs provide preprinted or computer-generated discharge instructions for particular problems; these should be used if available, because they undoubtedly will be more detailed than your own written instructions.

More than just discharge instructions must be carefully documented. ED notes tend to be brief and full of abbreviations, but keep in mind that they are medicolegal documents, just as all medical records are. Always document your thought processes, include pertinent positive *and* negative findings in your note, and write short continuation notes documenting repeat exams or responses to therapy. Remember the old adage, "not written means not done." You may be convinced that the 30-year-old with pleuritic right-sided sharp chest pain has no cardiac problems, but picture the scene in court after he drops dead of a heart attack, and your note is found to read: "30 male chest pain. Lungs clear. Heart RRR no m/g/r." Why didn't you order an ECG? Why were you so convinced his pain was noncardiac? Your notes should reflect this. Being concise does not mean being incomplete. A warning, though: Do not let your zeal for documentation disrupt patient care. Usually there will be ample time to complete notes after the patient is stabilized and the disposition is established. With time and practice you'll find that you can write better and better notes in less and less time.

At the beginning and end of each shift, you will go through a ritual handing-off of responsibility for patients, usually known as "sign-out." When you are leaving, it's a good idea to prepare for this. Check all of your patients' charts to ensure that you've written your note, make all the phone calls or consult calls you can (because you know the patient best), and make sure that the workup (labs, x-rays, etc.) is being carried out. Before signing out, walk by the rooms to check that you haven't forgotten a particular patient (yes, this happens!). At sign-out, make sure the oncoming person who will take over for your patient knows what has been done, what needs to be done, and what you think is going on with the patient. Conversely, when you are coming in, make sure you get all this information, and ask for it if you don't get it. Smooth sign-outs are vital for proper patient care and patient flow!

A few final notes: While you are working in the ED, what you wear and carry can make a difference in your ability to do your job. Clothing should be neat, clean, and functional. Avoid necklaces, dangling earrings, scarves, and ties (in most places); patients or visitors with behavioral problems may grab these, seriously injuring you in the process. Also avoid wearing anything of great value, such as an expensive watch or Grandma's ring. They could easily be damaged or stolen in the hectic environment of the ED. Always wear comfortable shoes—as an experiment, try wearing poorly fitting shoes for a shift and see how you feel!

Equipment you burden yourself with should serve a real purpose. In most cases you won't need a tuning fork or ophthalmoscope; the first is seldom needed, and the second is usually mounted on the wall in each room. A good stethoscope is vital, and it is the only piece of equipment many ED physicians carry. It can also double as a reflex hammer. A good pen light can be useful—even more so a working pen (but a cheap one, because it may very well end up permanently "borrowed"). A good pair of heavy-duty shears is quite helpful (so-called paramedic shears) for cutting bandages, clothing, and so on. Index cards to keep track of each patient will help you to keep your thoughts organized. Most important, bring your wits, enthusiasm, and energy—you will find them taxed but stimulated in the organized chaos of the ED.

2

Know Your ABCs: Resuscitation and Stabilization

The ABCs are just that! They form the basic approach to all patients in the ED no matter how trivial the presenting complaint seems. ABC stands for airway, breathing, and circulation. By performing a rapid assessment of these for every patient, you will minimize your chances of missing a life-threatening problem.

Although the ABCs are presented in a sequential manner in order of priorities, remember that emergency medicine is a team effort. Therefore, often all three aspects will be addressed simultaneously.

AIRWAY

We cannot overemphasize the importance of assessing and managing a patient's airway. Assessment begins as the patient enters the room:

- Is the patient able to talk?
- Is there hoarseness, stridor, or cyanosis?
- Are there any suprasternal, intercostal, or subcostal retractions?

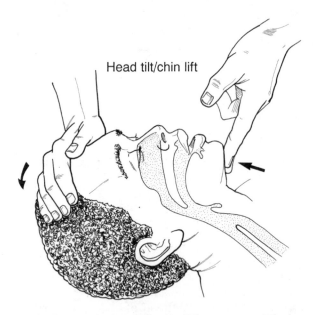

Head tilt/chin lift

Figure 2–1. The head-tilt/chin-lift maneuver. Tilt the head backwards with one hand, while the other hand lifts the chin forward.

- Are there obvious facial fractures, broken teeth, or particles of vomitus in the mouth?

The most common cause of upper airway obstruction in the supine unconscious patient is posterior displacement of the base of the tongue, usually in patients with an altered mental status. Therefore, start by opening the airway and bringing the tongue forward. This is best accomplished using a combined head tilt and chin lift (Fig. 2–1). When cervical spine (C-spine) injury is suspected, immobilize the neck (e.g., with a hard collar, head blocks) and perform a jaw thrust (Fig. 2–2). Avoid moving the neck. Open the mouth and look to see if there are any obvious causes of obstruction, such as broken teeth, dentures, foreign bodies, or

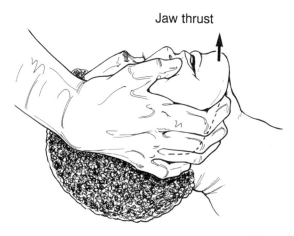

Jaw thrust

Figure 2–2. In the jaw-thrust maneuver, place your fingers behind the angle of the patient's jaw and forcefully bring it forward.

vomitus. Use a hard-tipped suction catheter to clean out the mouth. If the patient starts breathing more easily, you may want to insert an oral or nasopharyngeal airway, as tolerated by the patient.

Intubation

Patients with a compromised airway need definitive airway management by endotracheal intubation or establishment of a surgical airway. *As a rule, anyone who can tolerate it should be intubated.* Indications for intubation include:

- Apnea
- Airway obstruction
- Respiratory failure
- Risk of aspiration in a patient with an altered mental state
- Controlled hyperventilation in patients with

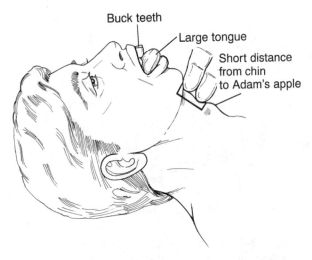

Figure 2–3. Anatomic features of a difficult airway.

severe head injuries, usually with a Glasgow Coma Scale (GCS) score < 8 (see Table 3–2)
- Control of the combative patient to avoid further injury

The decision to intubate should be made based on clinical grounds. Do not wait for ABGs or a chest x-ray. The biggest pitfall in airway management is failing to intubate the patient in a timely fashion.

Anticipating a Difficult Intubation

The following clinical parameters suggest that intubation will be technically difficult:

- A short neck
- Buck teeth
- A large tongue
- A short distance between the tip of the chin and thyroid cartilage (less than three finger breadths [Fig. 2–3])

If any of these are present, you may want to call for backup (e.g., an anesthesiologist) or attempt naso-tracheal intubation or fiberoptic laryngoscopy if the patient is breathing spontaneously.

Methods of Airway Management

Although most textbooks emphasize the technique of endotracheal intubation, it is important for you to spend time mastering the proper use of the bag valve mask (BVM). To be effective, it is often necessary for two people to perform BVM ventilation. The BVM enables both oxygenation and ventilation of the patient when you are unable to intubate the patient immediately, and it allows time to mobilize personnel more experienced in airway management. Remember, however, that the airway remains unprotected from aspiration when a BVM is used, and proper head positioning is required to minimize inadvertent ventilation of the stomach. The major difficulty when using the BVM is maintaining a good mask seal; therefore, the two-handed method is most effective (Fig. 2–4).

Rapid Sequence Induction Intubation

The most useful tool for emergency intubation is rapid sequence induction (RSI). In RSI, general anesthesia and neuromuscular blockade are induced to achieve optimum intubating conditions and patient control while maintaining maximum protection against aspiration. Always assume that the patient has a full stomach. Also, be prepared to establish a surgical airway if intubation is unsuccessful. The patient should not be ventilated with a BVM prior to the initial attempt to intubate. This

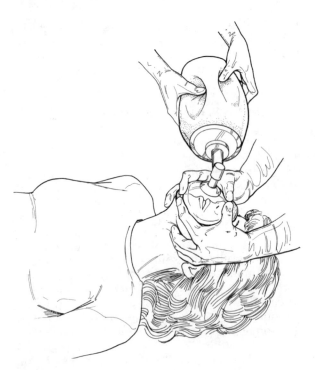

Figure 2–4. The two-handed technique: one rescuer achieves a tight two-handed seal with the mask, while the other rescuer squeezes the bag.

helps avoid gastric distention and passive regurgitation during the procedure.

The sequence of RSI may be remembered using the "Five Ps":

1. **Preoxygenate:** Give O_2 via a non-rebreather mask for 5 minutes. This builds an O_2 reserve that allows apnea for 3 to 5 minutes.
2. **Prepare the following:**
   a. Suction (hard-tipped Yankauer catheter in case of regurgitation).
   b. Two working IV lines.

   c. Monitors (cardiac, pulse oximeter, end-tidal CO_2).

   d. Laryngoscope (fresh batteries and bulb).

   e. Blades—a #3 or #4 Macintosh for most adults, a #2 Miller for children younger than 8 years of age, or a #1 Miller for infants.

   f. Endotracheal tubes: men, 7.0 to 8.5 mm; women, 6.5 to 8.0 mm. In children, the size of the endotracheal tube may be estimated by using the following formula:

$$\text{Tube size} = \frac{\text{Child's age} + 16}{4}.$$

   g. Stylet (this should not protrude through the end of the tube).

   h. BVM, connected to 100% O_2.

   i. Direct a nurse to draw up all drugs and label them appropriately.

   j. Have a cricothyroidotomy set available and opened.

   k. Patient positioning: align the oropharyngeal-laryngeal axis by placing the patient in the "sniffing" position (neck flexed, head extended). The patient's head should be raised 2 to 4 inches by placing a pad or a blanket under the head (Fig. 2–5). *Do not move the patient's head if cervical trauma is suspected.*

3. **Pretreat:** Lidocaine 1 mg/kg by IV push (IVP) may blunt the sudden rise in intracranial pressure (ICP) induced by laryngoscopy and intubation. Give vecuronium 1 mg IVP (0.01 mg/kg) as a defasciculating dose before using a depolarizing paralytic agent to avoid fasciculations.

4. **Induce and Paralyze**

   a. *Induce* with etomidate 20 mg IVP (0. ̃ kg), thiopental 350 to 5C ̃ mg/kg), or midazolam 5 ̦ mg/kg). You may omit in tient is comatose.

   b. *Paralyze* with either succin̦

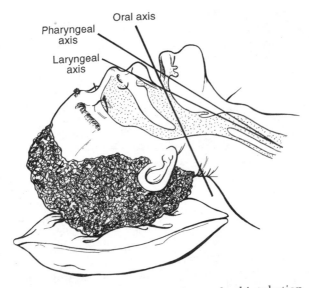

Figure 2–5. Head positioning for tracheal intubation. In the sniffing position the neck is flexed while the head is extended. This creates the shortest distance and straightest line between the mouth and the vocal cords.

    IVP (1.0 to 1.5 mg/kg) or vecuronium 10 mg IVP (0.1 mg/kg).
  c. *Perform the Sellick maneuver:* After giving the induction agent, have an assistant apply pressure with his or her thumb and index finger to the cricoid cartilage, thus compressing and occluding the esophagus against the C-spine to avoid passive gastroesophageal reflux and aspiration (Fig. 2–6). You should apply cricoid pressure at the onset of apnea and maintain it until endotracheal tube placement is confirmed. If active esophageal regurgitation occurs, you must release cricoid pressure.

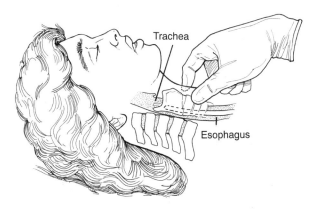

Figure 2–6. The Sellick maneuver: the thumb and index finger press down on the cricoid cartilage, compressing the esophagus against the spine.

5. **Pass the tube:** Proceed with intubation after confirming that the following conditions exist: apnea, lack of eyelid twitch upon stimulation, and flaccidity of the jaw. You should pass the endotracheal tube only after you see the true vocal cords or glottic aperture. Insert the blade of the laryngoscope into the right corner of the mouth and push the tongue to the left (Fig. 2–7). You should pull the handle of the laryngoscope in the direction that it points (90° to the blade). Avoid cocking the handle back, which may break the teeth. If you see the glottis but cannot advance the tube, have your assistant reduce the cricoid pressure. You may find Magil forceps helpful in this situation. Confirm tube placement by the following methods:
   a. Presence of breath sounds over both lungs (especially over the left axilla)
   b. Improved oxygenation
   c. Increasing end-tidal CO_2 (if available)
   d. Fogging of the tube
   e. A chest x-ray

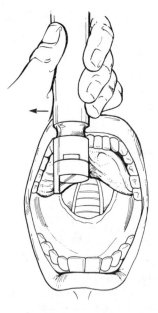

Figure 2–7. By inserting the laryngoscope in the right corner of the mouth, this pushes the tongue out of the way, allowing visualization of the cords and passage of the endotracheal tube.

Free aspiration of greater than 10 to 20 mL of air from the end of the endotracheal tube has been described recently as a simple and accurate method to verify placement in the trachea. After inflating the endotracheal tube cuff with 10 mL of air, release cricoid pressure and secure the tube with tape or umbilical cord. The end of the endotracheal tube should then be connected to a BVM or ventilator. At this point, you should consider giving additional sedation and/or paralysis as indicated. Oxygen saturation should be monitored by pulse oximetry during the procedure. Desaturation should be avoided. If you are unable to intubate, stop and manually ventilate the patient with a BVM before reattempting intubation.

Although it is important to be familiar with all the medications used in RSI (Table 2–1), it is easiest to remember one standard formula that is effective in the majority of cases:

1. Preoxygenate.
2. Prepare all equipment.
3. Pretreat with vecuronium (defasciculating dose = 1 mg).
4. Induce with etomidate 0.3 mg/kg IVP (rapid, short-acting, minimal myocardial and respiratory depression).
5. Paralyze with succinylcholine 1.5 mg/kg IVP (rapid, short-acting).
6. Intubate and confirm tube placement.

Modification of the standard sequence of RSI should be made in the following conditions:

- **Increased ICP:** Pretreat with lidocaine and fentanyl (3 µg/kg IVP) to blunt the increase in ICP with laryngoscopy and intubation.
- **Status asthmaticus:** Use ketamine (1 mg/kg IVP), which has direct bronchodilatory effects and leads to release of catecholamines, for induction.
- **Congestive heart failure (CHF):** Avoid myocardial depressants, such as thiopental and succinylcholine. Etomidate and vecuronium are good alternatives.
- **Status epilepticus:** Induce with thiopental, which suppresses epileptogenic foci and increases the seizure threshold.
- **Blunt multiple trauma:** Patients often are hypotensive; therefore, etomidate, which causes minimal myocardial depression, is the preferred induction agent. *Be aware that as you intubate a hypovolemic patient and ventilate with positive-pressure breathing, right ven-*

Table 2-1. DRUGS USED IN RAPID SEQUENCE INTUBATION

MEDICATION	DOSE (MG/KG)	ONSET (MIN)	DURATION (MIN)	COMMENTS
Etomidate	0.2–0.3	1	4–10	Nausea, vomiting, myoclonus, adrenal suppression, cardiac depression; agent of choice in trauma and CHF
Thiopental	3.0–5.0	1	10–30	Hypotension, histamine release; decreases ICP
Midazolam	0.1–0.2	1	30–80	Minimal adverse effects; can be given IM
Ketamine	1.0	1	15–30	Emergent hallucinations, increased BP, bronchodilation
Succinylcholine	1.5	<1	4–6	Bradycardia, hyperkalemia, masseter muscle spasm, malignant hyperthermia, increased ICP; contraindicated in penetrating eye injuries
Vecuronium	0.1–0.2	1–2	4–6	Minimal adverse effects
Pancuronium	0.05–0.10	3	40–60	Lower dosage in renal failure; vagolytic

BP = blood pressure; CHF = congestive heart failure; ICP = intracranial pressure; IM = intramuscularly.

tricular filling may be impeded, resulting in a decrease in the systemic blood pressure (BP). Treat this with fluids and minimization of high airway pressures, continuing sedation or paralysis as required.

BREATHING

Assessment

After ensuring an open airway, assess whether the patient is breathing adequately. Look for signs of chest wall movement and symmetry. Feel and listen for air movement. Auscultate with a stethoscope for bilateral breath sounds. The patient in respiratory failure may be tachypnic, cyanotic, speechless, or lethargic. Paradoxic abdominal breathing (inward abdominal movement with inspiration), as well as suprasternal, subcostal, and intercostal retractions, all are evidence of respiratory distress. Look for signs of a tension pneumothorax (tracheal deviation away from the side of decreased breath sounds, jugular venous distention). If the patient is not breathing adequately, assist patient ventilation with a BVM or a ventilator.

Ventilators

Pressure cycled respirators usually are used in infants weighing less than 10 kg, whereas volume cycled respirators are used in larger patients.

Initial ventilator settings may be estimated with the following formulas:

1. Tidal volume (TV): 10 to 20 mL/kg.
2. Respiratory Rate (RR): 12 to 16 breaths per minute (faster in a patient with suspected increased ICP).

3. F_{IO_2}: Start with 100%, and then adjust to maintain an O_2 saturation > 90%.

If the patient remains hypoxic despite 100% O_2, check if there is a pneumothorax. If none exists, consider adding positive end-expiratory pressure (PEEP) in increments of 2 cm H_2O. ABGs should be drawn within 10 to 15 minutes to ensure proper ventilation and oxygenation.

Ventilating the Severely Tight Asthmatic

Sometimes it is technically difficult to ventilate the patient with severe bronchospasm. Low tidal volumes should be used, and the RR should be adjusted to maintain adequate oxygenation (Pao_2 > 60). Hyperventilation should be avoided, however, because it can cause dangerously high airway pressures, with resultant barotrauma. High levels of CO_2 may need to be tolerated (permissive hypercapnea). Also, the inspiratory-to-expiratory ratio should be adjusted for a prolonged expiratory phase.

Interpretation of Arterial Blood Gases

It is beyond the scope of this book to review ABG analysis in detail, so we will provide only an overview. ABGs measure the following parameters:

1. **$Paco_2$**: This is a direct measure of ventilation. A $Paco_2$ < 35 means that the patient is hyperventilating. A $Paco_2$ > 45 means that the patient is hypoventilating. Note that some patients with chronic obstructive pulmonary disease (COPD) chronically retain CO_2, and in these patients the pH should be used to assess ventilation.
2. **Pao_2**: This is a measure of the adequacy of oxy-

genation. Calculating the alveolar-arterial oxygen gradient (A-a gradient) will help sort out the various causes of hypoxemia. For example, in a patient breathing room air at sea level, the alveolar Po_2 may be estimated by subtracting the $Paco_2$ from 145:

$$(\text{A-a gradient} = 145 - Paco_2 - Pao_2)$$

If the patient is on supplemental oxygen, the Pao_2 may be estimated by multiplying the Fio_2 by 6. The A-a gradient is then calculated by subtracting the Pao_2 from the Pao_2. Hypoxia with a normal A-a gradient (10–15) is rare, and it is caused either by hypoventilation or by a low alveolar Fio_2. Hypoxia with an increased A-a gradient is more common, and it usually is due to mismatched ventilation-perfusion (V/Q mismatch). Arteriovenous shunting or a diffusion barrier are other causes of hypoxemia with an increased A-a gradient. Failure of the hypoxia to respond to 100% O_2 suggests a right-left shunt.

3. **pH**: This defines the acid-base balance. Many disturbances are mixed. In pure acid-base disturbances, the relationships between pH, $Paco_2$, and HCO_3 can be estimated using the following formulas:

   a. In metabolic acidosis, the $Paco_2$ should equal 1.5 (HCO_3) + 8.
   b. In metabolic alkalosis, the $Paco_2$ should equal 0.9 (HCO_3).
   c. In respiratory acidosis, the HCO_3 should increase by 1 mEq/L for every 10-mm Hg increase in $Paco_2$.
   d. In respiratory alkalosis, the HCO_3 should fall 2 mEq/L for every 10-mm Hg decrease in $Paco_2$.

If the changes in $Paco_2$ or HCO_3 differ significantly from the expected compensatory changes, a mixed acid-base disturbance should be suspected.

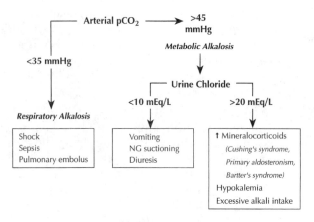

Figure 2–8. The differential diagnosis of alkalemia.

Figures 2–8 and 2–9 present a useful approach to the differential diagnosis of acid-base disturbances.

CIRCULATION AND SHOCK

The circulatory system is composed of a *pump* (the heart), *fluid* (the blood), and a system of *tubes* (blood vessels). Its sole purpose is to supply vital nutrients (e.g., oxygen, glucose) to the tissues and to return waste products (e.g., carbon dioxide) for elimination. Shock is defined as a state of circulatory insufficiency, whereby perfusion is inadequate to meet the metabolic needs of the cells.

The major pitfalls in shock management are the failure to recognize circulatory insufficiency in its earlier states, awaiting a drop in the arterial BP before diagnosing shock, and insufficient fluid resuscitation.

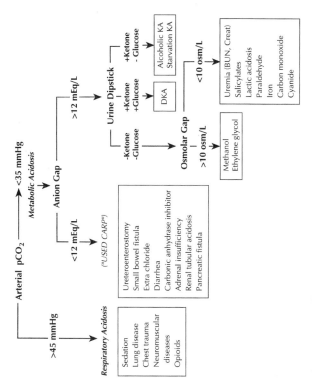

Figure 2–9. The differential diagnosis of acidemia.

Etiology of Shock

Ultimately, shock management requires recognition and correction of the underlying cause. The following are the more common causes of shock seen in the ED according to mechanism:

- **Hypovolemic shock** (failure of fluids) is the most common cause of shock seen in the trauma patient and is usually due to blood loss. Other causes of hypovolemic shock include diarrhea, vomiting, and overzealous diuresis.
- **Cardiogenic shock** (pump failure) is due to abnormalities of chronotropy (both rapid and slow heart rates) or inotropy (systolic or diastolic myocardial dysfunction).
- **Distributive shock** (failure of tubes) is due to redistribution of the fluids within the circulatory system, resulting in inadequate flow. This type of shock includes septic, neurogenic, and anaphylactic shock.

Assessment of Shock

Shock is characterized by a low flow state (an extreme state of shock is seen in cases of cardiac or traumatic arrest, where there is no flow at all). Therefore, tissue perfusion should be assessed, not just the BP. Assess tissue perfusion by examining the following clinical parameters:

- **Pulse:** After assessing the airway and breathing, check for a pulse. The peripheral pulse usually will be lost when the systemic arterial BP falls below 70 to 80 mm Hg; therefore, you should start by assessing a central pulse at the carotid or femoral arteries. If no pulse is palpable within 5 to 10 seconds, proceed with external cardiac massage (cardiopulmonary resuscitation [CPR]). Place the heel of your nondominant hand over the lower part of the sternum and compress 2 to 4 inches at a rate of 80 to 100 times per minute. Do not forget to assess periodically for spontaneous resumption of the pulse and respirations. If a central pulse is palpated, check a peripheral pulse for the following characteristics: (1) Is it rapid? (you don't have to count the heart rate to know that it is too fast!); (2) Is it weak and thready?

- **Central nervous system (CNS):** One of the earliest signs of shock is agitation. As the systemic arterial BP falls below 80 mm Hg, the patient becomes confused and ultimately loses consciousness.
- **Skin:** As blood is shunted away from the skin to preserve cerebral and cardiac circulation, the skin becomes cool and clammy. In the past, much emphasis was placed on capillary refill as a good indicator of peripheral perfusion. However, more recent studies have failed to validate its usefulness.
- **Cardiac:** In cases of severe shock, especially in patients with underlying coronary artery disease, the myocardium may become ischemic; the patient will complain of chest pain or shortness of breath and may develop a tachycardia.
- **Systemic BP:** Because of compensatory mechanisms (mainly sympathetic stimulation), supine BP usually is maintained until more than 20% to 25% of the blood volume is lost. Also remember that although a BP of 120/80 mm Hg often is felt to be normal, BPs vary widely. Therefore, do not rely on a single BP measurement to estimate the adequacy of circulation. Orthostatic changes in BP (a decrease of greater than 20 mm Hg in systolic BP) or pulse (an increase of 20 to 30 beats per

minute in the heart rate) usually indicate a 10% to 15% loss in blood volume. Subjective dizziness is probably the most sensitive indicator of orthostasis.

- **Renal:** Normal urine output is approximately 30 to 50 mL/h (1 mL/kg per hour in children). Decreased urinary output is an early sign of shock, so accurate assessment of urinary output is one of the cornerstones of shock evaluation and management.
- **pH:** The presence of metabolic acidosis suggests severe hypoperfusion and advanced shock.

DYSRHYTHMIAS

A detailed description of the various dysrhythmias is beyond the scope of this book; rather, we present a simplified approach to the unstable patient with an arrhythmia. Generally, to manage the unstable patient, you should be able to answer the following questions:

- Is there a pulse?
- What is the heart rate?
- Is the rhythm organized?

Figure 2–10 presents a simple approach to managing dysrhythmias in the unstable patient.

ARRESTS AND RESUSCITATIONS

Most patients who come into the ED *in extremis* are brought in by emergency medical services (EMS). Don't miss this opportunity to obtain vital information concerning the patient's present and

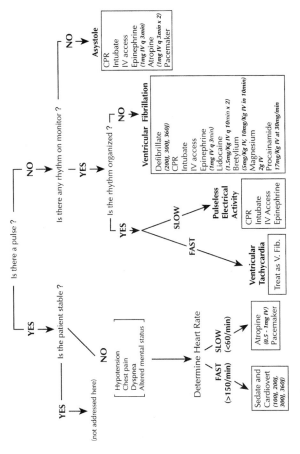

Figure 2–10. Approach to dysrhythmias.

29

past illnesses. Often the patient will be brought in without family members or friends, and this might be your only chance to obtain pertinent information concerning the patient. All the relevant information should be obtained briefly from the EMS crew while the patient is being wheeled into the room and transferred from the stretcher to the bed. Also don't forget that many EDs have telemetry capabilities and serve as EMS base stations; much vital information can be obtained even before the patient arrives at the ED.

The following information should be obtained from prehospital personnel before their departure from the ED:

- Time the patient was found unresponsive
- Presence and timing of bystander CPR
- Time until arrival of EMS and initiation of CPR
- Initial rhythm and vital signs
- Therapy given at the scene and en route, and the patient's response
- A brief description of the scene of arrest (evidence of trauma, overdose, etc.)
- Evidence and estimation of external blood loss
- Past medical history, medications, and allergies if known
- Presence of "Do Not Resuscitate" (DNR) orders, advance directives, health care proxy, or a living will

On learning about the imminent arrival of a patient *in extremis,* the following preparations will expedite the care of the patient on arrival:

1. Prepare an airway station—suction apparatus, laryngoscopy, endotracheal tubes, BVM, O_2.
2. Prepare IV access and fluids—large-bore (#14- or #16-gauge) angiocatheters and several bags of normal saline (NS) solution with tubing.

Also, have syringes, needles, and lab tubes available.
3. Notify backup teams as needed and required by the nature of the case (e.g., surgeons, anesthesiologists, respiratory therapists, pediatricians).
4. Determine the team leader and delegate responsibilities to the team members, such as IV access, airway management, defibrillation, medication administration, and documentation.
5. Dress for the occasion. Resuscitations, whether medical or traumatic, can be very messy (e.g., with blood, vomitus). Put on gloves, mask, goggles or face shield, water-resistant gown, and shoe covers before the patient's arrival.

Advanced Cardiac Life Support (ACLS) guidelines and treatment protocols appear in Appendix A. You are strongly encouraged to read the original recommendations in the October 28, 1992, issue of JAMA.

GENERAL RECOMMENDATIONS

The following general recommendations can help you avoid the more common mistakes and pitfalls in ED resuscitations:

1. Establish yourself as the team leader and discourage unnecessary noises and distractions. (Remember, however, that you will need help: You can't do everything yourself.)
2. Don't forget to apply "quick look" paddles first before establishing IVs, performing endotracheal intubation, etc.
3. If the patient is in ventricular fibrillation, apply three defibrillations as required, in rapid succession. Do not waste time checking for a pulse between *initial* defibrillations.

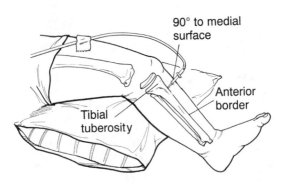

Figure 2–11. Intraosseous cannulation technique.

4. Initially, peripheral IV access should be obtained, but central venous access should be established as soon as practical because central drug administration has been shown to be more effective than peripheral administration. In children, if IV access is not obtained within 60 seconds, intraosseous access should be performed at the midanterior tibia (Fig. 2–11).

5. Don't forget to defibrillate the patient 30 to 60 seconds after each drug is administered for ventricular fibrillation. After drug administration, flush the line with 10 to 20 mL NS to facilitate its distribution.

6. Continuously reassess the patient for the presence of a pulse and spontaneous respirations. Endotracheal tube placement and the patient's color also should be re-evaluated.

7. Don't forget to give magnesium 2 g IV for resistant ventricular fibrillation.

8. Transcutaneous pacing in patients with bradycardia or asystole, when readily available, is extremely useful.

9. If pulseless electrical activity is present, attempt to rule out underlying conditions, such as:
   a. hypovolemia (give a fluid bolus)

b. tension pneumothorax (perform bilateral needle thoracostomies)
c. pericardial tamponade (perform pericardiocentesis)
d. acidosis (correct ventilation and administer bicarbonate for a pH below 7.1)
e. hyperkalemia (give calcium chloride and bicarbonate)

3

Trauma

GENERAL PRINCIPLES

In no other situation is it more important to perform a rapid and thorough assessment than in the multiply injured patient. Your goal is to identify and initiate management for those salvageable injuries that can cause death (if unrecognized) during the first "golden hour." Emergency medicine is a team effort. Although the assessment and management of the multiply injured patient will be presented in a sequential manner in order of priority, in the clinical setting multiple steps should be addressed simultaneously.

Patient management consists of a rapid primary evaluation, resuscitation of vital functions, a more detailed secondary evaluation, and finally, the initiation of definitive care.

History

Trauma can be divided into two major types: *blunt* and *penetrating.* Blunt trauma is often multiple and occult, whereas penetrating trauma is usually more limited and readily apparent. Therefore, patients with blunt trauma have greater mortality and morbidity secondary to a delay in diagnosis.

Ascertaining the mechanism of initial trauma can help you predict the types and severity of resulting injuries. Each type of trauma injury is associated with a distinct set of circumstances. Therefore, one must gather all of the following relevant information:

- **Motor vehicle accidents:** Direction of impact; appearance of vehicle (body, windshield, steering wheel, and column); use of restraining devices, seat belts, and/or air bags; and estimated speed at impact (remember energy equals mass times velocity squared). Ejection of the patient from the vehicle or the death of another passenger significantly increases the likelihood that the patient has serious injuries. Also, try to estimate the degree of external blood loss at the scene.
- **Falls:** From what height and onto what type of surface did the patient fall?
- **Penetrating trauma:** Where was the patient injured? What weapon was used? What was the estimated distance of the patient from the weapon? What was the velocity and caliber of the bullet?

Other important information that should be considered in your evaluation include damage to structures surrounding the trauma victim at the scene, extrication problems, injuries suffered by others in the same event, events preceding the injury, recent alcohol or drug use, and last oral intake of food or beverage. A history of prior illnesses, surgeries, medications, immunizations, and allergies also should be obtained.

THE PRIMARY SURVEY:
ASSESSMENT OF THE ABCDEs

During this stage, you must recognize life-threatening conditions and initiate management simultaneously. Once a problem is identified, it must be addressed before proceeding to the next stage.

Airway and Cervical Spine

Cervical spine (C-spine) injuries are present in approximately 1% to 2% of all blunt trauma patients and in 5% to 10% of patients with head trauma. However, it is safest always to assume a C-spine fracture is present. Excessive motion of the unstable C-spine (both hyperextension and hyperflexion) can cause further neurologic damage. Recent studies in cadavers demonstrate that all methods of airway management result in movement of the C-spine.

Rapidly assess the upper airway for obstruction (see Chapter 2). Use the chin lift and/or jaw thrust to establish airway patency. Look in the mouth for foreign bodies, debris, and vomitus. If the airway is compromised, RSI with inline C-spine immobilization is the preferred method of airway control.

The following is a summary of RSI in the patient with head injury:

1. **Preoxygenate** with 100% O_2.
2. **Pretreat** with vecuronium (0.01 mg/kg IVP), lidocaine (1.5 mg/kg IVP), and fentanyl (3–5 µg/kg IV).
3. **Induce** with etomidate (0.3 mg/kg IVP, with multiple injuries) *or* thiopental (3 to 5 mg/kg IVP in isolated head injuries).
4. **Paralyze** with succinylcholine (1.5 mg/kg IV).

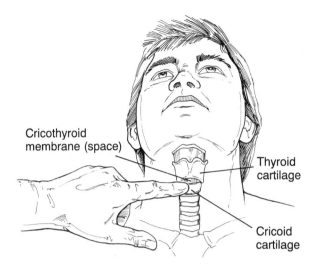

Cricothyroid
membrane (space)

Thyroid
cartilage

Cricoid
cartilage

Figure 3–1. Cricothyroid membrane anatomy.

5. **Perform orotracheal intubation** with C-spine immobilization.

For a more detailed discussion of RSI, refer to Chapter 2.

Surgical Airways

If you are unable to intubate the patient because of obstructive lesions, you must perform needle or surgical cricothyroidotomy through the cricothyroid membrane. You can find this membrane by locating the suprasternal notch and advancing your finger cephalad in the midline. The first hard cartilaginous structure you encounter is the cricoid cartilage. The soft cricothyroid membrane is immediately above this and below the thyroid cartilage ("the Adam's apple," Fig. 3–1).

Needle cricothyroidotomy is performed by inserting a large-bore angiocatheter attached to a 10-mL syringe through this membrane at a 45° angle

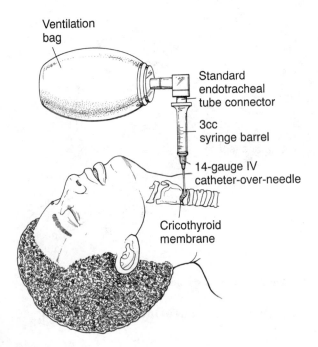

Ventilation
bag

Standard
endotracheal
tube connector

3cc
syringe barrel

14-gauge IV
catheter-over-needle

Cricothyroid
membrane

Figure 3–2. Needle cricothyroidotomy.

in the caudal direction. Aspirating for air while advancing can help avoid cannulation of the esophagus or the soft tissues. The hub of the angiocatheter should be connected to a 3-mm endotracheal tube adapter or to a 3-mL syringe and 7.5 mm adapter, which will enable ventilation with the use of a BVM, or a jet insufflator at a pressure of 50 pounds per square inch (psi) (Fig. 3–2). This method should be used only as a temporizing agent because it usually will result in hypercarbia after 30 minutes.

Surgical cricothyroidotomy is the definitive surgical airway. A midline superficial vertical incision is made between the suprasternal notch and the thyroid cartilage. After the cricothyroid membrane is identified, a horizontal incision is made through it by gently puncturing it with the tip of a #11 blade. This opening then is enlarged with a surgical clamp, and a 6-mm endotracheal tube (or specialized tracheostomy tube) is inserted between the spread ends of the clamp (Fig. 3–3). Surgical cricothyroidotomy should be avoided in children younger than 8 years old because of their small airways.

Breathing

During this stage, you should attempt to identify three traumatic conditions that most often compromise ventilation: (1) tension pneumothorax; (2) open pneumothorax; and (3) large flail chests with an underlying pulmonary contusion. Examine the chest and assess for adequacy of air exchange:

- Is the chest wall moving?
- Is the movement symmetric?
- Are there any obvious injuries (e.g., open wounds, contusions, abrasions)?

Auscultate below the armpits bilaterally for the presence of breath sounds:

- Is the trachea midline?
- Is there jugular venous distention?
- Is there paradoxic motion of a flail segment of the chest?

If you suspect a tension pneumothorax (i.e., respiratory distress, absent breath sounds, deviated trachea and mediastinum, elevated central venous pressure, poor peripheral perfusion) insert a #18- or #16-gauge angiocatheter attached to a fluid-filled syringe in the second intercostal space at the midclavicular line. The appearance of air bubbles in the fluid-filled syringe both confirms and de-

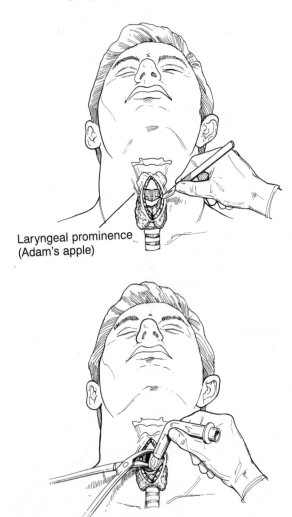

Laryngeal prominence
(Adam's apple)

Figure 3–3. Surgical cricothyroidotomy.

compresses a pneumothorax (remember that the patient will need a more definitive chest tube placed after you complete your primary survey). If you find an open chest wound an occlusive dressing should be placed immediately. If one is already in place, or if on placing an occlusive dressing the patient's respiratory status suddenly deteriorates, remove the occlusive dressing and insert a chest tube before reapplying an occlusive dressing.

All trauma patients should receive supplemental 100% O_2 via a non-rebreather mask or a BVM.

Circulation

Significant external bleeding should be identified and controlled during the primary survey by direct manual pressure on the wound. Do not blindly insert surgical clamps in wounds in an attempt to stop bleeding. Peripheral perfusion is assessed by examining the patient's level of consciousness, pulse, BP, skin, urine output, and ABGs.

Hemorrhagic shock secondary to acute blood loss is the most common cause of shock in trauma patients. However, other causes of shock should always be considered, especially if the patient is not responding to treatment. *Cardiogenic shock* may be due to underlying cardiac disease or may be the result of a cardiac contusion or pericardial tamponade. *Neurogenic shock* should be considered in patients with relative bradycardia and warm skin. *Hypovolemic shock* is divided into four stages of increasing severity based on the degree of blood loss. Table 3–1 a useful classification of shock based on the percentage of volume lost, the average blood loss, and the presence of clinical parameters.

Early recognition of the shock state, aggressive fluid management, and identification and correc-

Table 3–1. CLASSIFICATION OF HYPOVOLEMIC SHOCK

	CLASS OF SHOCK			
	1	2	3	4
Blood volume loss	<15%	20–25%	30–35%	>40%
Signs and symptoms	None	Postural only	Postural symptoms, decreased urine output, hypoperfusion, acidosis	Hypotension, anuria
Average blood loss (mL)	500	1000	1500	>2000
Whole blood lost (U)	1	2	3	>4
Crystalloid requirements (mL)	1500	3000	4500	6000

tion of the underlying cause are the cornerstones of management. In many trauma patients, this means getting them to the operating room as soon as possible.

Intravenous Access

Intravenous access must be established as soon as possible with at least two large-bore peripheral IVs (#14- or #16-gauge angiocatheters). Central venous catheters are not part of the initial resuscitation unless no other access is available. They may play an important diagnostic and monitoring role later in the management, but they rarely are required during the primary survey.

The following are sites for IV access *in order of preference* (remember that this is not the time to save the "best" veins for last to demonstrate your skills as a phlebotomist):

1. **Antecubital veins,** which usually are easy to visualize or palpate.
2. **Other peripheral upper-extremity veins** in the forearm or hand. The cephalic vein, located over the lateral radial aspect of the wrist, often is a good choice.
3. **Saphenous venous cut down.** Perform a 2-cm horizontal incision, 1 cm anterior and 1 cm proximal to the medial malleolus at the ankle. Isolate the greater saphenous vein by blunt dissection with a curved hemostat and cannulate with a large-bore angiocatheter (Fig. 3–4).
4. **The femoral vein,** which is located medial to the femoral artery distal to the inguinal ligament. If no pulse is palpable, insert the needle distal to the inguinal ligament one finger breadth medial to the halfway point between the anterior superior iliac spine and the pubic tubercle (Fig. 3–5). An 8F catheter should be in-

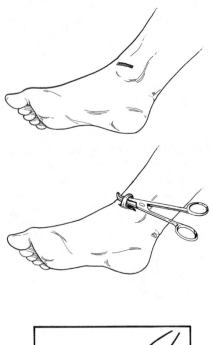

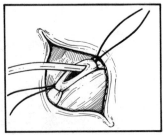

Figure 3–4. Saphenous venous cutdown.

troduced into the vein over a wire. This may be faster and easier than a saphenous venous cutdown.
5. **Subclavian or internal jugular vein,** whichever you are more comfortable with. Use an 8F short catheter.

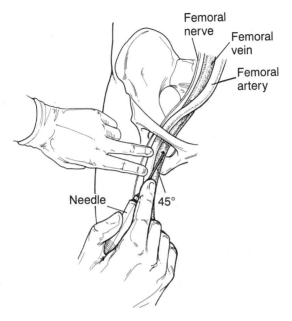

Figure 3–5. Femoral vein cannulation.

Fluids

Although the issue of crystalloids vs. colloids is controversial, crystalloids should be the initial choice in shock. Either NS or lactated Ringer's solution may be used. As a rule, three times as much crystalloids are required to replace the loss of a given amount of blood. Begin by giving a 2-liter fluid bolus as rapidly as possible (rapid infusion pumps are available in some emergency departments). Further fluid management will be determined by the response to this initial fluid challenge. If the patient remains hypotensive, give blood. Although type-specific blood is preferable (usually available within 10 minutes), type O-negative blood should be given if the patient is hemodynamically unstable.

Blood usually is given as packed red blood cells (PRBCs). Generally, give 2 U of fresh frozen plasma for every 6 U of PRBCs transfused. With very rapid infusion of blood, both platelets and calcium chloride may be required. Note that blood products must be diluted with NS, not lactated Ringer's solution.

Disability

During the primary survey, a brief neurologic evaluation, including level of consciousness and a pupil examination, should be performed.

1. **The patient's level of consciousness** may be described using the **AVPU** method:

   A—alert
   V—responds to *vocal* stimuli
   P—responds to *painful* stimuli (pain should be applied above the clavicles, such as supra-orbital pressure)
   U—unresponsive to all stimuli

   The GCS has no place in the primary survey; it is used during the secondary survey. However, if the patient is to be intubated and paralyzed, rapid GCS assessment is essential for the neurosurgeon. Often it is enough to say, "Open your eyes," and note the response to noxious stimuli, such as IV attempts.

2. **Pupils**: Look at the pupils. Note their size. Are they equal? Do the pupils react to light? Pupillary inequality or unresponsiveness may be a sign of increased ICP, resulting in uncal herniation and pressure on the third cranial nerve nucleus on the side of the larger pupil. Note that in the normal population, 10% to 15% of people have anisocoria, in which the pupils do respond to light.

Exposure

Completely undress the patient and remove all garments and jewelry. Now is not the time to be modest. All nooks and crannies must be assessed. After completing your assessment, cover the patient with a warm blanket. It is easier to prevent hypothermia than to treat the resulting complications.

Monitoring

All patients in shock should be connected to a cardiac monitor and pulse oximetry. An automated BP monitor or an arterial line should be placed. If the patient remains hypotensive, consider inserting a central venous pressure catheter to assess for elevated right-sided pressures that may be caused by pericardial tamponade or for very low pressures that require more aggressive fluid or blood resuscitation.

RESUSCITATION

Although presented separately, resuscitative efforts should be instituted while the primary and secondary surveys are being performed.

The following elements should be part of the resuscitation of all trauma patients:

- **O$_2$:** All patients should receive supplemental O$_2$ via a non-rebreather mask or a BVM.
- **IV access:** All patients should have at least two peripheral large-bore IVs established, as described in the previous section in this chapter on IV Access (i.e., in patients in hypovolemic shock). When inserting an IV, blood

should be drawn immediately for type and cross-match as well as for a baseline CBC, chemistry, and amylase. Seriously injured patients should have a spun hematocrit (for more details on how to spin a "crit," see Chapter 11). If you insert an angiocatheter and have difficulty obtaining the required amount of blood, draw blood from the femoral artery to avoid wasting precious time.

- **Urinary output** should be monitored after an indwelling urethral catheter is placed. Attempts should be made first to obtain a spontaneously voided urine because urethral catheterization can cause injury and some bleeding. Always examine the genitalia and perform a rectal exam before inserting a urethral catheter. Contraindications to urinary catheterization include blood at the external meatus, perineal or scrotal hematoma, and a high-riding or nonpalpable prostate. If a urinary catheter cannot be placed, the patient will need an emergent retrograde urethrogram.

- **Gastric catheters** should be considered at this point. Aspiration of blood suggests gastrointestinal injury. Emptying the stomach also reduces the risk of aspiration and relieves pressure on the diaphragm that can limit adequate ventilation. In cases of significant nasal trauma or suspected skull fracture, an orogastric tube should be placed (because of the risk of a nasal approach leading to intracranial intubation). Early placement of a gastric catheter also enables administration of oral contrast when an abdominal computed tomographic (CT) scan is required.

- **A radiologic trauma screen** should be obtained, including a cross-table lateral view of the neck, a supine anteroposterior view of the chest, and a pelvic view. Usually it is easiest to film all three areas in rapid succession before having the technician develop the films. All other x-rays should be performed after stabilization and performance of a more detailed secondary survey.

THE SECONDARY SURVEY

Only a brief summary of the secondary survey will be presented. Several often-neglected areas will be highlighted.

Head

Even when the neck is immobilized, it usually is possible to insert your hand beneath the head and carefully palpate for areas of swelling, bleeding, or irregularity. If the patient is alert, try to assess visual acuity. Ask the patient to read your name off your ID badge. Do a quick visual confrontation exam. If a corneal injury is likely, stain the eye with fluorescein and observe it under a portable Wood's lamp. If you have difficulty opening the eye because of swelling, paper clips bent in two can be used to create eyelid retractors.

Look in the nares for evidence of blood or cerebrospinal fluid (CSF). Epistaxis should be tamponaded with the use of a nasal tampon. Observe the nasal septum for a hematoma using an otoscope and attached adult earpiece. Septal hematomas should be drained with a #18-gauge needle or a #11 blade.

Look into the ears for blood, CSF, or a hemotympanum (blood behind the eardrum). A hemotympanum is the most common clinical finding in basilar skull fractures.

Table 3–2. THE GLASGOW COMA SCALE

1. BEST VERBAL RESPONSE

None	1
Incomprehensible sounds	2
Inappropriate words	3
Confused	4
Oriented	5

2. EYE OPENING

None	1
To pain	2
To command	3
Spontaneously	4

3. BEST MOTOR RESPONSE

None	1
Abnormal extension	2
Abnormal flexion	3
Withdrawal	4
Localizes	5
Obeys commands	6

Total Score	**3–15**

Central Nervous System

At this point, a determination of the patient's level of consciousness based on the GCS should be made. Check eye opening, verbal response, and motor response to stimuli of increasing intensity (Table 3–2). The best responses should be used to calculate the GCS. Complete a full motor and sensory evaluation of the extremities. (If the patient is unconscious, a sensory exam is obviously omitted.) The patient's neurologic status should be reassessed continually (every 10–15 minutes) for any signs of deterioration.

The degree of brain damage is determined by primary insults at the time of injury (e.g., laceration, contusion) and by secondary insults from ischemia and edema. Therefore, it is vital to recognize and aggressively treat elevations in the ICP as early as possible to avoid any further injury to the brain.

The *sine qua non* of increased ICP with herniation is unconsciousness. ICP with herniation is suggested by the following signs and symptoms:

- GCS < 8.
- Unequal pupils (anisocoria > 1 mm) in a patient with an altered mental status
- Cushing's triad (hypertension, bradycardia, and abnormal respirations)
- Deteriorating neurologic status
- Significant edema or midline shift visualized on a head CT scan
- Lateralizing neurologic signs

The following measures will help decrease ICP:

1. Intubate and hyperventilate the patient *down* to a $Paco_2$ of 25 to 30 mm Hg by ventilating the patient 20 to 25 times per minute (once the $Paco_2$ drops below 25 mm Hg, significant cerebral vasoconstriction will occur and cause a decreased perfusion pressure that can cause more ischemic damage).
2. Elevate the head of the bed to 30° if shock has been corrected.
3. Give mannitol 1 g/kg IV rapidly (avoid in the hypotensive patient).
4. Sedate the patient; give morphine sulfate 0.1 mg/kg IV every hour.
5. Paralyze the patient; give vecuronium or pancuronium 0.1 mg/kg IV every hour.
6. Maintain normothermia. (If patient is febrile, give antipyretics.)

Indications for a head CT scan in the multiply injured patient include:

- Head injury with skull penetration
- Any alteration in the level of consciousness
- A clear history of substantial loss of consciousness with memory deficit
- Focal neurologic findings or lateralization on exam
- Recurrent vomiting
- Increasing headache

Any patient with significant signs or symptoms suggesting intracranial injury should be admitted for observation and possibly a repeat head CT scan in 24 hours, even if the initial CT scan is negative.

Maxillofacial Trauma

Palpate for areas of tenderness and instability. Grasp the upper teeth and assess for midface instability. Have the patient open and close his or her mouth and assess for malocclusion.

Cervical Spine

At this point most patients have their neck immobilized with a hard collar. Insert your hand beneath the neck, palpating for tenderness, swelling, or instability. Have an assistant manually stabilize the neck while the collar is removed. Absence of pain or neurologic deficit does not rule out C-spine injury.

A cross-table lateral film of the neck will identify 80% to 90% of cervical fractures. Adding an anterior-posterior film of the neck and an open-mouth view (odontoid film) will help identify most other C-spine injuries. However, if you still suspect injury, additional films or scans of the neck (e.g., oblique, flexion-extension, CT, or magnetic resonance imaging [MRI]) may be performed. Remember that a C-spine injury can be ruled out only if all seven vertebrae, including the C7 to T1 alignment, are visualized. To facilitate visualization of the lower vertebrae, pull down on the patient's arms while obtaining the cross-table lateral film. If either of the arms is injured, wrap a long sheet around the shoulder from front to back and apply traction in the direction of the feet. If you still cannot see all the cervical vertebrae, a "swimmers" view is recommended.

Ruling Out a C-Spine Injury in the Clinical Setting

No x-ray is indicated if the patient fulfills all of the following criteria:

- The patient is alert.
- The patient is not intoxicated.
- There are no significant distracting injuries (i.e., an extremity fracture).
- There is no midline neck tenderness.
- The patient denies having any neck pain.

If a C-spine series is not indicated based on the above criteria, remove the cervical collar and ask the patient to move his or her head (e.g., nod yes, nod no, touch ear to each shoulder). If the patient performs all the above without significant discomfort, no x-rays are indicated and you may safely leave off the cervical collar.

Chest

Visualize the chest in its entirety. Palpate the entire chest wall for areas of tenderness, instability, and subcutaneous emphysema. Feel both clavicles and each rib individually. Listen for heart sounds, their regularity, and the presence of murmurs and

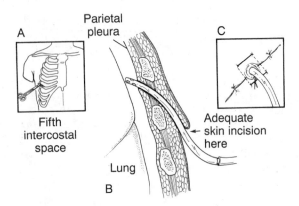

Figure 3–6. Chest tube placement. (*A*) Location of chest tube insertion. (*B*) Tunnel the tube through the subcutaneous tissue and above the rib superior to the site of insertion. (*C*) Secure the tube with a purse string suture.

gallops. Auscultate for breath sounds high on the anterior chest (for pneumothorax) and at the posterior bases (for hemothorax). Distant heart sounds and distended neck veins may indicate cardiac tamponade (in the presence of hypovolemia, however, neck veins may not be distended). Indications for chest tube placement include:

- Penetrating trauma to the chest: Don't forget that high abdominal and flank injuries can also invade the pleural cavity.
- Hemothorax or pneumothorax.
- Subcutaneous emphysema and multiple rib fractures, especially if the patient is to be taken to the operating room and ventilated with positive pressure.

If a chest tube is indicated, use a large chest tube (#34 Fr) and insert the tube anterior to the midaxillary line at the level of the fifth intercostal space (at the level of the nipple in men or at the level of the inframammary fold in women) (Fig. 3–6*A*).

Prep and drape the chest at the site of insertion and, if time allows, locally anesthetize the skin and rib periosteum with 1% lidocaine. A horizontal 2- to 3-cm incision should be made over the rib below the predetermined space. Then bluntly dissect through the subcutaneous tissues over the top of the rib, and carefully puncture the parietal pleura with the tip of a large clamp. Insert your finger into the incision, and to avoid further injury, perform a 360° sweep, feeling for organs (lungs, heart, liver, spleen) and adhesions before inserting the chest tube.

Because most trauma patients have a combined pneumothorax and hemothorax and are usually supine, direct your chest tube posteriorly, superiorly, and medially. Make sure all side holes are within the pleural cavity. Look for condensation in the chest tube. Do not let go of the tube until it is adequately secured with a #0 silk or mersilene suture and adhesive tape (Fig. 3–6*C*). The end of the chest tube should be attached to an underwater seal apparatus and suction (-20 cm H_2O) or a Pleuravac. Verify tube placement and function by obtaining a stat chest x-ray.

Abdomen

Focus on determining whether an abdominal injury exists and if surgical intervention is required. Frequent reassessments will help you identify any change in the patient's condition. The abdominal examination involves the following:

- **Inspection:** Are there any obvious penetrating injuries or evisceration of intra-abdominal organs (which usually are absolute indications for operative intervention)? (Some institutions are selective in cases of stab wounds.) Are there any significant abrasions or contusions indicating injury? Is the abdomen distended?

- **Auscultation of the abdomen:** This rarely is useful because most trauma patients will have an ileus.
- **Palpation for areas of tenderness, rigidity, or masses:** Always perform a rectal exam for evidence of obvious rectal tears, pelvic fractures, or blood. Note the rectal tone and the position of the prostate gland.

Diagnostic Aids

The use of peritoneal lavage vs. abdominal CT scan in abdominal trauma is controversial. The initial choice of either technique varies from institution to institution based on the clinicians' experience, immediate availability and quality of CT scanning, and reliability of radiologic interpretation. If a new-generation CT apparatus and good radiologic backup are immediately available, CT scanning might be chosen first. It often gives more specific anatomic information and allows assessment of the retroperitoneal space as well. Some institutions use sequential peritoneal lavage together with CT scanning. Recently there also has been an increase of bedside ultrasound for identifying fluid in the abdomen. If the patient is too unstable to be transferred to the CT scanner, peritoneal lavage should be chosen.

Indications for peritoneal lavage or abdominal CT scanning (with oral and IV contrast) include:

- Equivocal abdominal findings (e.g., in the presence of fractured ribs or lumbar spine fracture)
- The presence of head injury, intoxication, or paraplegia, which make the abdominal exam unreliable
- When the patient requires other lengthy evaluations or surgery (which precludes frequent reassessment)

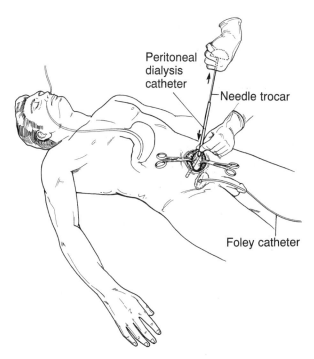

Peritoneal
dialysis
catheter

Needle trocar

Foley catheter

Figure 3–7. Peritoneal lavage. An assistant should place traction on the transversalis fascia and peritoneum.

- The presence of unexplained hypotension

If you choose to perform a peritoneal lavage, we suggest you use a semiopen technique with an incision through the skin and subcutaneous tissue before inserting a peritoneal dialysis catheter over a trocar. Have an assistant apply traction and elevate the abdominal wall with a pair of clamps. This will make using the peritoneal trocar easier and safer. Usually, peritoneal lavage should be performed below the umbilicus in the midline (Fig. 3–7). Always decompress the stomach and bladder with a gastric tube and urinary catheter before performing lavage to avoid damage to these organs. Aspirate for blood or obvious enteric contents. If none are present, instill 1 liter of warm crystalloid (10 mL/kg in children) and then drain by gravity.

The following findings on peritoneal lavage usually indicate the need for exploratory laparotomy:

- \> 5 mL of gross blood on aspiration
- Obvious enteric contents (food, feces)
- Appearance of peritoneal fluid in urinary catheter or chest tube
- \> 100,000 RBCs/mL of peritoneal lavage fluid
- \> 500 white blood cells (WBCs)/mL of peritoneal lavage fluid
- Amylase > 175 U (controversial)

Peritoneal lavage and/or abdominal CT scanning should never be performed when early surgical intervention is clearly indicated, such as in the hemodynamically unstable patient with evidence of abdominal trauma or in the patient with unequivocal peritoneal irritation.

Pelvis

It is important to identify pelvic fractures because they often are associated with other injuries, such as damage to blood vessels with resulting retroperitoneal hemorrhage. Anteroposterior and lateral compression should be applied to the pelvic ring, assessing for the presence of tenderness, instability, or obvious deformities. Urine should be obtained for a urine dipstick which, if negative, reliably rules out hematuria. Remember that a positive dipstick may also be caused by hemoglobinuria (usually pink) or myoglobinuria (usually cola-colored). Therefore, if the dipstick is positive, send urine for microscopic analysis to confirm the presence of hematuria. Isolated microhematuria in the hemodynamically stable patient does not need further workup. In female patients, a digital vaginal exam for the presence of blood or fractures must be performed. Priapism in men suggests spinal cord injury. Arteriography with embolization often is required to treat retroperitoneal hemorrhage.

Extremities

All extremities should be inspected for swelling, ecchymosis, or obvious deformities. All peripheral pulses should be assessed. If pulses are not palpable, try using a portable Doppler. Emergent arteriography should be considered in the presence of an arterial bleeder, an expanding hematoma, or a penetrating trauma in proximity to a major blood vessel.

Palpate all bones with rotational or three-point pressure for tenderness, crepitus, or abnormal movement. Obvious fractures or dislocations with loss of distal pulses should be reduced as early as is feasible. (Try to rule out C-spine injury and give analgesics before reduction).

Log roll the patient as a unit while immobilizing the head and neck, and inspect and palpate the thoracic and lumbar spine for areas of swelling, deformity, or tenderness. Don't forget to look between the buttocks for evidence of injury.

GENERAL RECOMMENDATIONS

The following is a summary of general recommendations based on our experience and common pitfalls in managing the multiply injured patient:

1. Assign a team leader and delegate responsibilities. Often members of multiple disciplines

will be present (usually responding to a trauma code). If possible, preassign the different roles of the team members before the patient arrives. The team leader usually is the most senior member and is responsible for performing the primary and secondary survey and overseeing the performance of all other team members. One team member (preferably with an assistant, such as a respiratory therapist) is responsible for airway management and breathing. Another member should be responsible for obtaining IV access. Assign a team member to the perineal region. His or her responsibility is to draw all the necessary blood (including ABGs) from the femoral artery, perform a rectal exam, and if not contraindicated, insert a urethral Foley catheter.

2. Don't forget to <u>log roll</u> the patient.
3. Always assume a C-spine injury before proving otherwise.
4. Always perform a rectal exam before inserting a urinary catheter.
5. Don't forget to perform a digital vaginal exam in female patients, looking for blood and evidence of a pelvic fracture.
6. If a patient fails to stabilize after rapid crystalloid infusion, give blood.
7. Don't delay the transport of an unstable patient to the operating room to complete physical, radiologic, or lab assessment (all may be completed in the operating room).
8. Continually reassess the patient's vital signs, airway, and endotracheal tube placement.
9. Don't forget to palpate and document all extremity pulses.
10. Most multiply injured patients will need the following "trauma screen:" chest x-ray, C-spine films, pelvic x-ray, blood type and cross, CBC, glucose and electrolytes, blood urea nitrogen (BUN), creatinine, prothrom-

bin time (PT) and partial thromboplastin time (PTT), amylase, urinalysis, ECG, and ABGs.

11. Never presume that hypotension is caused by a head injury.

12. Don't be afraid to push fluids in patients with head or spinal cord injuries who are hemodynamically unstable.

13. Avoid overly aggressive fluid resuscitation in the hemodynamically stable patient with head or spinal cord injuries.

14. Always get a rectal temperature. Hypothermia should be avoided and aggressively managed.

15. Consider using tetanus prophylaxis and antibiotics (see Chapter 15 on Wound Management).

4

CHAPTER

Chest Pain

Chest pain is a very common chief complaint in most EDs. It can indicate disease ranging from the benign to the immediately fatal. In the evaluation of chest pain, the patient's history is *vitally* important. Physical examination and adjunctive tests can be helpful, but they often will be normal, as in many cases of myocardial ischemia. Our concern is that we do not miss the diagnosis of serious cardiac, vascular, or respiratory disorders such as myocardial infarction or unstable angina, new angina, pulmonary embolism (PE), or an aortic dissection.

HISTORY

When taking the patient's history, focus your questions on the character of the pain (e.g., sharp, dull), the time course of the pain, whether it is worsened by respiration (i.e., the pain is "pleuritic"), and what alleviating or aggravating factors there are. Pleuritic pain usually indicates a noncardiac etiology, such as costochondritis, pneumonia, or pneumothorax. Cardiac pain usually is not affected by the respiratory cycle, although pericarditis can give rise to pain that is aggravated by deep inspiration or a supine position. Also, ask about any recent chest trauma. Inquire about associated symptoms, such as cough and fever (think of pneumonia), or palpitations, nausea, shortness of breath, and diaphoresis (think of cardiac disease). Ask about cardiac risk factors: hypertension, diabetes, smoking, high cholesterol, sedentary lifestyle, or cardiac disease that developed in a first-degree relative younger than 50 years of age. Also, ask about recent use of cocaine, which can cause myocardial ischemia, often with an atypical presentation.

PHYSICAL EXAMINATION

The physical exam should focus on the lungs and cardiovascular system. Listen for decreased breath sounds, wheezes, rubs, or rales. Murmurs or gallops may direct you to cardiac disease. Look for signs of CHF, such as peripheral edema, jugular venous distention, or hepatomegaly. Examine the chest wall as well, looking for localized tenderness, ecchymosis, or rash (such as zoster). All patients with other than obviously benign chest pain should be placed on a cardiac monitor and pulse oximetry. To enable rapid drug administration in the event that a dysrhythmia should develop, IV access should be established before you conduct a comprehensive H&P.

ANCILLARY TESTS

The tests of importance usually are the ECG and chest x-ray. In general, order an ECG for any patient with chest pain in whom you cannot absolutely exclude cardiac disease. Order a chest x-ray and pulse oximetry (or an ABG) for any patient with pulmonary signs or symptoms (especially chest pain or dyspnea), or in whom you suspect pulmonary disease. Patients with probable cardiac disease also should have an x-ray to look at heart size and the presence of CHF. Every chest x-ray should be evaluated for the presence of a widened mediastinum (greater than 6 to 8 cm), suggesting aortic dissection, and pneumomediastinum, suggesting esophageal rupture.

Earlier and more sensitive and specific markers of myocardial injury (such as CPK-MB, myoglobin, and troponin I) are playing a more crucial role in the early decision-making process in the ED. When the results of such tests are readily available, a negative test should never dissuade you from admitting a patient with a history suggestive of myocardial ischemia.

DIFFERENTIAL DIAGNOSIS

Certain causes of chest pain, as discussed below, are so potentially dangerous that you must consider and exclude them for every patient with this complaint. Often these problems will have characteristic H&P findings, and the summary below should help you in sorting these out. Table 4–1 also includes some key points.

Aortic Dissection

Classically, patients with aortic dissection describe their pain as a sudden tearing, located in the mid or left chest or in the upper back. They often have a history of hypertension or have used drugs (e.g., cocaine) that can cause hypertension. De-

Table 4-1. DIFFERENTIAL DIAGNOSIS OF CHEST PAIN

ETIOLOGY	ONSET/COURSE	QUALITY	LOCATION/RADIATION	EXACERBATING FACTORS
Angina	Rapid/brief	Pressure	Chest, neck, arms	Exertion, stress
Myocardial infarction	Rapid/>30 min	Pressure	Chest, neck, arms	Stress or none
Aortic dissection	Sudden/severe	Tearing	Chest and back	Hypertension
Pulmonary embolism	Sudden	Sharp, pleuritic	Chest, back	Deep breath, cough
Esophageal rupture	Sudden/severe	Sharp, burning	Chest, throat, back	Swallowing, vomiting
Pericarditis	Gradual	Sharp, pleuritic	Precordium	Supine position
Musculoskeletal	Variable	Sharp, dull	Localized	Movement

pending on which arteries have been disrupted by the dissection, they may have neurologic deficits or unequal pulses or BPs in the extremities. If the dissection has compromised the coronary circulation, they can have the signs and symptoms of myocardial ischemia or infarction. The aortic valve can be damaged, leading to aortic regurgitation. The valve may be wide open so that there may not be a murmur. The dissection can also rupture into the pericardium, causing cardiac tamponade.

If you suspect dissection, the initial treatment is to lower the BP with IV nitroprusside (0.5 to 10.0 µg/kg per minute) and beta-blockers (labetolol IV in incremental boluses starting at 20 to 40 mg), or with trimethaphan (1 to 4 mg/min). You then should order definitive diagnostic tests. In many institutions, this consists of an aortogram; others use MRI, contrast chest CT scanning, or transesophageal echocardiography. Our current practice is to get an aortogram in all patients in whom we strongly suspect this diagnosis, and to use chest CT scanning as a screen in stable patients who may have a dissection. Patients with proximal dissection will require surgery; those with distal dissection usually can be managed medically.

Pulmonary Embolism

In patients with a PE, chest pain may be pleuritic in nature or dull, mimicking a myocardial infarction (MI). These patients often complain of associated dyspnea. They may have hemoptysis. A history of immobility (e.g., a long plane flight), CHF, any underlying malignancy, or the use of cigarettes or birth control pills may be suggestive of PE. A history of prior deep-vein thrombosis or a PE should significantly raise your index of suspicion. Physical examination may reveal tachypnea or tenderness and swelling in the legs. Less than half of patients with a PE will be tachycardic. Therefore, you cannot rely on tachycardia to diagnose a PE. The ECG most commonly shows nonspecific ST-T changes or an $S_1Q_3T_3$ pattern. The chest x-ray may be normal, or it may show the classic "Hampton's hump" of pulmonary infarction (a wedge-shaped, pleural-based density) or Westermark's sign (increased central vascular markings with peripheral oligemia). An elevated hemidiaphragm is seen in half of PE cases. Blood gases usually show an increased A-a gradient and desaturation; 10% of patients may, however, have a totally normal blood gas.

The treatment for PE is IV heparinization, which should be started immediately if the diagnosis is strongly suspected, even before further diagnostic testing. An IV bolus of 80 U/kg followed by a continuous infusion of 18 U/kg per hour should be given and adjusted to achieve a PTT 1.5 to 2 times the normal.

The diagnosis can be established by an abnormal lung V/Q scan or by pulmonary angiography. There are only two options for a V/Q scan: it can be either normal or abnormal. The diagnosis of a PE is excluded in the patient who has a low clinical suspicion and a normal V/Q scan. If the scan is abnormal in any way (i.e., low or intermediate probability), the patient will need further tests to exclude a PE. Only the patient with high clinical suspicion and a high-probability scan should be treated for a PE without further studies. Noninvasive studies of the legs, looking for deep vein thrombosis, also can be useful. In most cases, we start with lung scanning, followed by leg studies if the scan is nondiagnostic. If the leg studies are negative but we still strongly suspect PE, we then get a pulmonary angiogram. The diagnostic approach to PE is summarized in Figure 4–1.

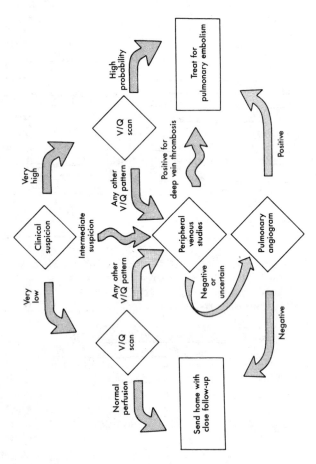

Figure 4–1. Approach to suspected pulmonary embolism. (From Feied C: Pulmonary Embolism. In Rosen P, et al. [eds], Emergency Medicine, ed 3, St Louis, 1990, CV Mosby Co., p 1304, with permission.)

Pneumothorax

Patients with pneumothorax usually complain of sharp and pleuritic chest pain, often with associated dyspnea. Often they are young, thin men. The lung exam may not show any abnormality, but the chest x-ray usually is diagnostic. It is sometimes helpful to get an end-expiratory film, which accentuates the abnormality. Treatment usually involves placing a chest tube or a smaller "pigtail" catheter into the pleural space. A word of warning: If the pneumothorax is under tension, the patient is likely to be in serious trouble. This entity should be diagnosed and treated *before* you get the chest x-ray. Suspect tension pneumothorax in a patient with hypotension, tracheal deviation, jugular venous distention, and unilaterally decreased breath sounds. The treatment of pneumothorax is discussed in Chapter 3.

Esophageal Rupture

Patients with esophageal rupture usually complain of severe midchest pain following repeated bouts of vomiting. Physical exam usually is not helpful, but the patient may have a fever. Chest x-ray may show pneumomediastinum or a pleural effusion. This diagnosis must be made expeditiously; delay in diagnosis of more than 12 hours is associated with extremely high mortality because of the onset of mediastinitis. Early surgical consultation is mandatory. IV antibiotics should be given as soon as the diagnosis is established.

Myocardial Ischemia or Infarction

These are put together because for the emergency physician there is no difference in the disposition. Classically, these patients complain of dull or heavy substernal chest pain. Anginal pain usually is initiated by activity, whereas the pain of infarction usually begins when the patient is resting. Patients may have a history of cardiac disease or risk factors. Physical exam often will be normal. Even the ECG will be normal or nonspecific in about one half of patients with ischemia, so this diagnosis often hinges on history alone.

Treatment of angina involves the use of nitrates (nitroglycerine 0.4 mg sublingually (SL) every 5 minutes, or nitropaste 1 to 2 inches to chest wall, or IV nitroglycerine 10 to 200 µg/min titrated to a 10% to 30% reduction in BP or pain relief) and aspirin 81 to 325 mg PO. In a patient with possible ischemia, without ECG evidence of infarction, morphine 2 to 5 mg IV may be useful for pain that does not respond to nitrates. Our usual procedure is to treat the patient with a nitroglycerin tablet SL every 3 to 5 minutes to a total of three tablets, and then if pain persists and the ECG is nondiagnostic, to treat the pain with morphine. In this case, you *must* repeat the ECG in about 30 minutes to 1 hour to see if new and diagnostic changes have developed. Treatment of an actual MI often requires the use of thrombolytics (streptokinase 1,500,000 U IV or t-PA 100 mg IV), IV nitroglycerin, IV beta-blockers (metoprolol 5 mg IV every 5 minutes to a total of 15 mg), or cardiac catheterization with emergent angioplasty or coronary artery bypass. Beta-blockers should be avoided in patients with cocaine-associated chest pain. Thrombolytic therapy is usually given if the ECG shows ST elevation of 1 mm or more in two or more contiguous leads, if the pain has lasted less than 12 hours. Before giving thrombolytics, be sure to ask the patient about contraindications, including active ulcer disease, surgery within the past 6 weeks, brain tumors or metastases, history of hemorrhagic stroke, bleeding disorders, or allergic reaction to thrombolytics, especially streptokinase. Patients with severe uncontrolled hypertension should have their BPs controlled before thrombolytics are given.

DISPOSITION

Most patients with chest pain will be admitted to the hospital. You should only discharge patients who have a clear and nondangerous etiology for their pain. Despite emergency medicine's best efforts, approximately 5% of patients with MI are sent home inadvertently each year. If you practice with the mind-set that every chest pain is a potential MI and that each patient must prove to you that coronary artery disease is not responsible for this pain, you will minimize your miss rate. With MIs, you often do not get a second chance to correct the mistake.

Several additional points merit comment:

- All chest pain is serious until evaluated fully.
- A blood gas never substitutes for a V/Q scan.
- A single ECG never excludes ischemic heart disease or an acute MI.
- Obtain a posteroanterior and lateral chest x-ray whenever possible. It will give you appropriate information about the mediastinum and heart size as well as the lung parenchyma.
- Patients younger than 30 years with no drug use (e.g., cocaine) with sharp, pleuritic, completely reproducible chest pain and a normal ECG are the only category of patients that you may safely discharge home nearly 100% of the time.
- There is no difference between an acute MI and a patient with unstable angina as to disposition.

5

Shortness of Breath

As with chest pain, dyspnea can reflect numerous diseases of varying severity. This chapter will outline some of the important aspects of working up the patient who is short of breath, but the discussion will not be exhaustive by any means. The protocols we give below reflect our practice; workup and treatment may vary in other hospitals.

A useful mnemonic for acute dyspnea is **PPOPPA:**

P = pulmonary embolus (PE)
P = pulmonary edema
O = obstruction (foreign body, epiglottitis, etc.)
P = pneumothorax
P = pneumonia
A = asthma or COPD

HISTORY

For many of these conditions, the patient's history will give important clues. Patients with asthma usually will be aware of their condition. A history of prior need for intubation or steroids in an asthmatic patient suggests a more severe prognosis. Inquire about cough, fever, or other associated symptoms. Is there orthopnea or paroxysmal nocturnal dyspnea? Is there a history of pedal edema? Ask about the risk factors for PE (see Chapter 4). Question the patient about exposure to tuberculosis and his or her purified protein derivative (PPD) status. Ask what medications the patient is taking. A long history of cigarette smoking suggests either COPD or lung cancer. Remember that not all that wheezes is asthma. All "new" asthmatics should be worked up for other causes.

PHYSICAL EXAMINATION

Physical examination can be very helpful. Fever usually is due to an infection but can appear with PE and many other disorders (e.g., MI, cancer). The lung exam is of course paramount, but don't neglect the cardiac exam, including looking for lateral displacement of the point of maximal impulse, jugular venous distention, and pedal edema, all of which suggest CHF. When examining the lungs, listen for rales, wheezes, bronchial breath sounds, decreased aeration, and egophony. Localized wheezes in the appropriate setting are suggestive of a bronchial foreign body. Percuss for dullness, and evaluate fremitus. Listen for stridor, as this is a very worrisome finding; it indicates some degree of upper airway obstruction. You should also beware of patients with "silent lungs" who do not have wheezes or rales. These patients are much sicker than most.

ANCILLARY TESTS

For patients with a history of asthma or COPD, bedside measurement of peak flow can be useful, especially if the patient's usual values are known, to gauge response to therapy. Normally, peak flows are in the range of 5 to 15 mL/kg. In addition, the advent of pulse oximetry has provided a quick, cheap, and noninvasive way to evaluate lung function. O_2 saturation should be measured for every patient with dyspnea. Be aware, though, that the reading only tells you about oxygenation and not ventilation (for which you need the CO_2 tension from a blood gas). Also, patients can have a "normal" saturation (e.g., 94%) and still have a substantially low blood O_2 tension (in this example, perhaps 66) and therefore a major A–a gradient. In any patient who has an abnormal pulse oximeter reading (below about 95%), or in whom you suspect moderate to severe lung disease, check an ABG.

The most important other diagnostic test is the chest x-ray. All dyspneic patients should have a chest x-ray unless they have diffuse wheezing that clears with therapy. In patients with chronic lung disease, try to get old films for comparison. Other tests to consider include an ECG, if cardiac disease is suspected, or the PE workup (see Chapter 4 for more details). Patients with fever and possible pneumonia should have blood cultures sent to rule out pneumococcal pneumonia.

DIFFERENTIAL DIAGNOSIS

One diagnostic dilemma you may face in the older dyspneic patient is differentiating between CHF and COPD. Both conditions can produce wheezing, but the therapies are markedly different. Sometimes the history will help, especially the patient's current medications. A chest x-ray often is extremely helpful. In cases where the film shows mild CHF but the patient's exam is more consistent with COPD, consider a trial of bronchodilator therapy. There is one caveat, however: it usually is a good idea to get an ECG first to rule out acute ischemia or MI; giving such patients beta-agonists may not be such a good idea because these drugs increase myocardial O_2 demand. Try to get old records or obtain results of prior stress tests or other cardiac workups to help you sort things out. If you are still unsure, and the patient is hemodynamically stable, you can try giving nitroglycerin SL to reduce preload. This will help in CHF but usually not in COPD.

TREATMENT

Several conditions present frequently enough or have such stereotyped treatment that we will now discuss our approach to them. In all cases we assume that the patient does *not* require intubation. The use of a CPAP (continuous positive airway pressure) mask can prevent the need for intubation. You may also use CPAP in patients who are retaining CO_2.

Asthma

Measure respiratory rate, heart rate, and peak flow, and assess the patient's color and use of accessory muscles of respiration. Use these variables to monitor the patient's response to therapy after each intervention. Begin treatment with nebulized beta-agonists. We use albuterol 2.5 mg in adults and children older than 5 years of age (1.25 to 2.5 mg in younger children) repeated every 20 minutes as long as no cardiovascular problems ensue. Aminophylline may be used, but we tend to avoid it because of its high potential for toxicity and low clinical added benefit to beta-agonists. If used, give an IV bolus of aminophylline 6 mg/kg, followed by a drip at 0.8 mg/kg per hour. Patients usually should have a chest x-ray done if they have fever, focal lung findings, first-time wheezing, or significant sputum production. After a total of three treatments over the course of 1 hour, re-evaluate the patient.

If there has been a steady improvement in the patient's dyspnea, respirations, and peak flow, and the patient has a peak flow greater than 70% of predicted value for age and height, discharge the patient on a short course of oral steroids, such as prednisone 40 mg/per day for 5 days in an adult. Usually no taper is needed after a short course such as this.

If the peak flow remains below 40% of the predicted value, give the patient IV corticosteroids (such as methylprednisolone 2 mg/kg to a maximum dose of 125 mg) and admit to the hospital. Patients with severe asthma and increasing CO_2 levels may need to be intubated. Intubation sometimes can be avoided in severe cases if you administer beta-agonists systemically (epinephrine 0.03 mg subcutaneously [SC]) or IV magnesium sulfate 2 g over 20 to 30 minutes. If intubation is required, induction with ketamine is appropriate (see Chapter 2).

For patients with intermediate peak flow values, therapy usually involves discharge on oral steroids, but you should keep a low threshold for admitting any of these patients. Any patient with active asthma and a concurrent lung disease, such as pneumonia, should be admitted.

A note on COPD: The treatment often is the same, but add four puffs of ipratropium bromide with each nebulizer treatment, as COPD tends to respond well to this agent. You may use ipratropium for all patients with asthma or COPD. It is impossible to know which patients in these two groups will respond to this agent, so the best approach is to use it "across the board."

Anaphylaxis

Patients with anaphylaxis usually have a history of allergy to some substance known to them to trigger these attacks, such as bee stings or foods such as peanuts. They can present with severe facial swelling, stridor, wheezing, and hypotension. If treated rapidly, they usually will recover quickly. If the patient at any point requires intubation or develops hypotension, ICU admission is mandatory.

Usually, begin therapy for early anaphylaxis with epinephrine 1:1000 solution 0.3 to 0.5 cc SC (0.01 mg/kg SC in children). Follow this with 50 mg/kg IV diphenhydramine (1.0 mg/kg in children). Patients with wheezing may benefit from nebulized beta-agonists. Be cautious with epinephrine in any patient with suspected coronary artery disease, but remember that anaphylaxis can kill, so be prepared to use epinephrine.

Any patient who has no history of hypotension and who has no dyspnea or stridor following treatment may be given one dose of IV corticosteroids and discharged on oral corticosteroids (such as prednisone as outlined above for asthma in adults) and diphenhydramine (usually 25 to 50 mg every 6 hours for adults) for several days. Observe these patients for about 4 to 6 hours before discharge to ensure that they do not relapse before the steroids begin to take effect.

All other patients should receive IV corticosteroids and be admitted. An H_2-blocker, such as cimetidine 300 mg IV, may have additional benefit in severe cases. Hypotensive patients will require epinephrine 1:10,000 solution 1 to 10 mg **slow** IVP to reverse life-threatening shock. Fluids are also critical to reverse the shock state; up to 6 liters of Ringer's lactate may be required.

Pulmonary Edema

The treatment modalities for pulmonary edema can be summarized by the mnemonic **LMNOP:**

L = lasix (furosemide) IV one or two times the patient's usual dose, or 40 mg if the patient is not usually on the drug.

M = morphine, given in doses of 2 to 4 mg IV. Avoid respiratory depression.

N = nitroglycerin, often given IV; may be given SL every 2 minutes while the drip is being prepared. Start with 5 to 10 μg/min IV and increase by 5 μg/min every 3 to 5 minutes. Hypotension should be avoided.

O = oxygen; 100% O_2 should be given to all patients with pulmonary edema.

P = position. The patient should be, and will want to be, sitting up.

In general, start therapy in an upright position with O_2, IV furosemide, and nitroglycerin SL. If the patient does not improve, start IV nitroglycerin at a rate of 10 μg/min, titrating to a 10% to 30% decrease in the mean arterial pressure. Give small doses of morphine to anxious patients. Throughout the treatment, follow the patient's pulmonary status (e.g., by pulse oximeter), RR, and urine output (which may require bladder catheterization). Get an ABG, ECG, and chest x-ray early.

Most of these patients will be admitted to the ICU. Some may go to a monitored step-down unit, a few may be able to go to an unmonitored bed, and only stable chronic patients will be discharged home. Consider intubation if the patient is worsening clinically, has deteriorating mental status, or remains hypoxic, acidotic, or hypercarbic after 20 to 30 minutes of aggressive therapy. When available, a CPAP mask may be an effective treatment, avoiding intubation.

6

CHAPTER

Abdominal Pain

Abdominal pain is a very challenging symptom to work up in the ED because of the broad differential diagnoses. This chapter will not include a detailed discussion of the many entities that can cause abdominal pain; instead, it will focus on some of the more pertinent points in the workup. Most important is that you do not miss serious disease, even if you cannot specifically diagnose the problem immediately. Be aware that the usual presenting signs and symptoms may be altered or absent in children, the elderly, AIDS patients, and any patient on corticosteroid therapy or with a chronic condition. It is best to be conservative with these patients, and in all those in whom a specific diagnosis cannot be established.

HISTORY

The history is crucial to the diagnosis. Ask about the time course, character, and location of the pain, including whether it has changed in any of these variables over time. Associated symptoms such as nausea, anorexia, fever, diarrhea, vomiting, vaginal bleeding or discharge, and dysuria may be important. Inquire as to how food has affected the pain. Most people inappropriately associate any abdominal problem with whatever they ate last. Find out when the patient <u>last ate</u>; this will be important if surgery is necessary. Note any <u>alcohol intake or medications</u> (e.g., NSAIDs) that can cause abdominal irritation or disorders. Inquire about <u>previous surgery</u>, a<u>natomic abnormalitie</u>s, or a <u>history of aortic aneurysm</u>. Always ask any woman when her <u>last menstrual period bega</u>n and whether it was <u>normal</u> for her or irregular or unusual in some way. *Any woman of childbearing age is considered pregnant until proven otherwise.*

PHYSICAL EXAMINATION

The physical exam should establish whether the patient has "<u>an acute surgical abdome</u>n" (i.e., <u>peritoneal signs</u> such as <u>rebound, rigidity, or guarding</u>). When examining for rebound, be as gentle as possible. It is sometimes helpful to percuss other than at the site of tenderness and see if that causes an increase in discomfort. For all patients, the exam *must* include a <u>rectal</u> and <u>genitourinary</u> exam; a <u>pelvic</u> exam also must be performed in female patients. Also remember to do a complete <u>chest exam</u>; more than one person has been fooled by a lower lobe pneumonia presenting as upper abdominal pain. Always <u>percuss for tenderness at the costovertebral angle</u>s.

ANCILLARY TESTS

Labwork in general should include a <u>CBC</u>, <u>electrolytes</u>, <u>glucose</u>, <u>BUN</u> and <u>creatinine</u>, <u>amylase</u> or <u>lipase</u>, <u>liver enzymes</u> (possibly), and a <u>urinalysis</u>. All women of childbearing age must have a <u>preg-</u>

nancy test, even if they tell you they couldn't possibly be pregnant. Older patients and children younger than 2 who have upper abdominal pain should have a chest x-ray taken. An upright chest x-ray is the appropriate study to exclude free intra-abdominal gas; if the patient cannot sit or stand, get a left-lateral-abdominal decubitus film for this purpose (air will be outlined against the liver). Abdominal films are rarely useful unless you suspect obstruction, but occasionally they may be helpful in cases of renal and biliary-tract disease, in which you would be looking for abnormal calcifications. Further studies such as IV pyelography, ultrasound, or abdominal CT scanning are very diagnosis- and institution-dependent.

DIFFERENTIAL DIAGNOSIS

The following are some diagnoses to consider, by location:

- **Right upper quadrant (RUQ):** hepatitis, cholecystitis or biliary colic, right lower lobe pneumonia
- **Left upper quadrant (LUQ):** peptic ulcer, gastritis, left lower lobe pneumonia
- **Midepigastric:** ulcer, pancreatitis, dyspeptic syndromes
- **Right lower quadrant (RLQ):** appendicitis, cecal volvulus, gynecologic pathology, testicular torsion
- **Left lower quadrant (LLQ):** diverticulitis, colitis (infectious or inflammatory), gynecologic pathology, testicular torsion
- **Anywhere:** ischemic bowel, inflammatory bowel disease, diabetic ketoacidosis, gastroenteritis

Cholecystitis

Acute cholecystitis is almost always (95%) due to gallstones. Acalculous cholecystitis typically is found only in elderly or debilitated patients. Pain usually is of sudden onset, radiating from the RUQ to the back. There usually is associated anorexia, nausea, and vomiting. The patient's RUQ will be tender. Fever often is present after 1 to 2 days of pain, but rarely before. Similar pain lasting only a few hours is usually due to biliary colic (i.e., gallstone impaction and then passage), a precursor to acute cholecystitis. An inspiratory arrest on deep palpation below the right costal margin (Murphy's sign) is commonly found. Patients may, however, present without any fever or leukocytosis.

Ultrasound usually can demonstrate the presence of gallstones, but it is only 80 to 90 percent sensitive for acute cholecystitis (evidenced by gallbladder wall thickening and the presence of pericholecystic fluid). The test of choice to exclude acute cholecystitis is hepatoiminodiacetic acid (HIDA) scanning. This test is positive when the isotope is unable to enter the cystic duct to fill the gallbladder; if the gallbladder is visualized, acute cholecystitis is excluded.

Patients with acute cholecystitis require admission for IV antibiotics and surgery. Patients with pain typical of biliary colic, but without acute cholecystitis and whose pain resolves, may be discharged with a surgical follow-up arranged.

Hepatitis

Hepatitis usually has a subacute course of days to weeks. It can be caused by either toxic exposures (e.g., ethanol, acetaminophen) or viral infection. The patient may have jaundice, RUQ pain, anorexia, nausea, and/or a low-grade fever. Liver enzymes will be elevated. Liver function should be assessed by checking coagulation parameters (PT and PTT).

Patients with hepatitis may not require admission in all cases, but they do require at least close follow-up with an internist or gastroenterologist. Admission is indicated in the following circumstances:

- Fulminant hepatitis with encephalopathy
- Severe vomiting and diarrhea with severe dehydration requiring IV hydration
- PT prolonged > 3 seconds above normal
- Hypoglycemia
- Bilirubin > 20 mg/dL
- Age greater than 45 years
- Immunosuppression
- Uncertain diagnosis

Beware of the alcoholic with RUQ pain. These patients may have a low-grade fever, jaundice, and tender hepatomegaly. A thorough search for other infectious diseases, such as pneumonia, urinary tract infection (UTI), sepsis, meningitis, and subacute bacterial peritonitis (SBE) is required. Any such patient with an altered mental status, fever, encephalopathy, or increasing abdominal girth requires a peritoneal tap and evaluation for SBE.

Peptic Ulcer Disease

Patients with peptic ulcer disease or gastritis may present with epigastric or LUQ pain sometimes radiating to the back. Cigarettes and alcohol are strongly associated with these disorders. The pain usually is relieved with antacids. You must exclude active or severe bleeding (by checking for rectal occult blood, nasogastric aspirate, orthostatic vital signs, and hematocrit) and perforation (either by exam or by chest x-ray for free air).

Many patients with inferior wall MIs also may present with similar symptoms. It is imperative that all patients, especially those with cardiac risk factors, receive an ECG to check for cardiac ischemia.

If all of these problems are excluded, the patient may be discharged on antacids (to be given 1 and 3 hours after meals and before bedtime) and H_2-blockers (cimetidine 800 mg or ranitidine 150 mg twice daily) with close follow-up.

Pancreatitis

Pancreatitis usually is caused by alcohol, gallstone impaction, trauma, or drug toxicity (e.g., thiazide diuretics, pentamidine, steroids). Patients present with severe epigastric pain radiating to the back, and often nausea and vomiting. The epigastric area usually will be tender, and rebound tenderness and guarding may be present. In severe cases, the patient may be in shock. Serum amylase and lipase usually will be elevated.

All patients with pancreatitis should be admitted and receive IV fluid hydration and pain management. The use of a nasogastric tube to prevent vomiting and to rest the bowel is controversial. Additional laboratory tests that are helpful in determining the patient's prognosis include WBC count, lactic dehydrogenase (LDH), serum glutamic oxaloacetic transaminase (SGOT), calcium and glucose.

Appendicitis

Appendicitis patients classically present with crampy periumbilical pain, which over a period of 12 to 24 hours localizes to the RLQ and becomes steady and sharp as peritoneal irritation occurs.

These patients often will have anorexia and a low-grade fever. Beware, though: The classic presentation is rare in the very young, the very old, and pregnant women. Always maintain a high index of suspicion for this disease in any patient with abdominal pain (especially men), and observe them for several hours with repeated examinations if you are not sure. There are no sensitive tests that will diagnose appendicitis. Many studies suggest that anorexia is present in all cases and that the WBC count is usually elevated. These findings may be helpful when they are present, but they do not help exclude the diagnosis in their absence. Therefore appendicitis still remains a clinical diagnosis; with minimal suspicion, obtain a surgical consultation. In experienced hands, RLQ ultrasound can be very helpful in questionable cases. Patients with obvious peritoneal signs should be taken to the operating room without major delays.

Diverticulitis

Diverticulitis often is called "left-sided appendicitis," and patients present with symptoms very similar to those associated with acute appendicitis, although diverticulitis is more commonly associated with LLQ findings. Similar cautions apply. Generally consider this disorder in elderly patients with abdominal pain and fever. Patients should be admitted if they have complicated diverticulitis, where surgical intervention is necessary for abscess, perforations, fistulas, and obstructions.

Ischemic Bowel

Ischemic bowel is also more common in the elderly, who often have atherosclerotic disease, and in patients who are predisposed to thrombosis. It typically presents as <u>pain out of proportion with physical findings</u>. Although abdominal x-ray may (rarely) show "thumbprinting" of the bowel wall, this diagnosis is hard to establish because most of the lab findings are nonspecific (elevated WBC or amylase) or late (acidosis). In elderly patients with abdominal pain, maintain a high index of suspicion for this disease and pursue it aggressively by ruling out other diseases and getting an <u>early surgical consultation</u>. Beware of the elderly patient with <u>atrial fibrillation</u>, in whom emboli may be thrown to the mesenteric arteries.

Gastroenteritis

Gastroenteritis is a common discharge diagnosis for patients with abdominal pain for whom no etiology was determined. Be aware, though, that the cardinal symptoms of this disease—usually due to a viral infection—are <u>vomiting and diarrhea</u>. In the <u>absence of these symptoms</u>, it usually is <u>better to discharge the patient with the diagnosis of "abdominal pain of unknown cause,"</u> rather than giving all concerned the false security of an erroneous diagnosis. All such patients should be <u>closely followed up</u>. Many disorders can cause nausea and vomiting (from glaucoma to intestinal obstructions), so it is essential that these patients be fully evaluated.

MANAGEMENT

<u>All patients with an "acute abdomen" (i.e., rebound, guarding, rigidity) should have an immediate surgical consultation</u>. Other patients with abdominal pain should have a <u>period of observation</u> in the ED unless a clear nonsurgical etiology for

the pain is found, or the pain resolves over the course of the ED visit. If the pain persists, an early surgical consultation can help expedite the disposition of many patients with abdominal pain. It is better to involve the surgeon earlier rather than later. Many surgeons prefer that patients do not receive pain medications before their exam, although some data exist showing that medication may actually improve the exam (by making the patient more comfortable and cooperative). This is a matter best discussed with your consultants to see what they prefer.

Unless a clear and benign diagnosis is made, it is safe to discharge patients with abdominal pain only if they appear well, can tolerate oral fluids, and can be reliably observed at home by a companion (who would be able to summon help if necessary). For these patients, detailed warnings and instructions should be given and close follow-up arranged.

7
CHAPTER

Neurologic Problems

COMA

The comatose patient often is very frightening even to experienced medical personnel. We hope that the following simple guidelines for the initial management of coma patients will make you more comfortable handling them. Our approach is a general framework; it may need to be altered in specific circumstances.

The initial approach to an unconscious patient differs from the traditional clinical assessment technique. Even *before* all the information about a patient is known, one may have to:

1. Stabilize basic life functions (ABCs)
2. Protect the patient from further harm
3. Promptly treat reversible disorders

The initial phase of resuscitation should follow the ABC format. Ensure that the patient has an open airway and is breathing; this may require intubation. Assess oxygenation by pulse oximetry, and give supplemental O_2 as necessary. Look for and treat hypotension if necessary. Obtain IV access and draw blood for the lab. Do an immediate chemstrip test for glucose if this is available. Give 2 mg of naloxone and 100 mg of thiamine IV. If the bedside glucose reading was low, or if you cannot perform that test, give 50 mL of 50% dextrose in water ($D_{50}W$) IV (in children 4 mL/kg of $D_{25}W$ IV). At this point, assuming you have successfully treated the abnormalities noted during your primary survey, you can go on to a more detailed evaluation.

History and Physical Examination

Whatever history can be obtained is vital. Question the people who found or brought in the patient about the circumstances in which he or she was found.

- Were any convulsions noted?
- Did the patient complain of anything before collapsing?
- Were any drugs, toxins, or alcohol found nearby or known to be available?
- What medical history is known?
- What is the patient's baseline mental status?
- Was there a rapid or progressive change in mental status?
- Is there any deterioration since they first saw the patient?
- Was there any evidence of trauma?

Do a general physical exam, looking especially for fever or rashes (consider meningococcemia or meningitis), needle marks (IV drug use), oral burns (toxic ingestion), nuchal rigidity, or signs of trauma (e.g., hemotympanum). Perform a rectal exam to look for occult blood. The neurologic exam should assess the following:

- **Respiratory pattern (if possible):** Apneustic or ataxic breathing indicates a brain stem injury, whereas Cheyne-Stokes breathing indicates bilateral hemispheric disease.
- **Pupillary reactivity and extraocular movements:** Also perform the cold-caloric test: Look into the ears to exclude tympanic membrane perforation; then instill 15 to 30 mL of

ice water into each ear canal while watching the eyes. The normal brain stem will drive the eyes slowly toward this stimulus, and the normal hemispheres will then cause nystagmus away from the stimulus. Hence, a patient with bilateral hemispheric injury or disease, such as in cases of poisoning or hypoxia, will show only a slow movement toward the ice water; the unresponsive patient has suffered damage to the brain stem, which usually is structural in nature (Fig. 7–1).

- **Motor tone:** Look especially for asymmetry of tone, which would indicate a localized structural lesion. Look also for decorticate or decerebrate posturing (Fig. 7–2).

Calculate a GCS score (see Chapter 3) on every patient. If the patient has to be sedated, paralyzed, or intubated, attempt to assess these variables very quickly before that intervention. All this requires is saying to the patient, "Open your eyes! What's your name?" and observing the response to supraorbital pressure or other noxious stimuli (one that works very well is the insertion of a cotton swab into the posterior nasopharynx). The GCS has some prognostic use for a patient who may require neurosurgical intervention.

The mnemonic **AEIOUTIPS** will help you remember the various causes of coma.

A = alcohols and ingested drugs and toxins
E = endocrine abnormalities and electrolyte disorders
I = insulin deficiency (diabetes)
O = oxygen deficiency and opioids
U = uremia
T = trauma
I = infection
P = psychiatric and porphyria
S = stroke, shock, subarachnoid hemorrhage, and space-occupying tumors

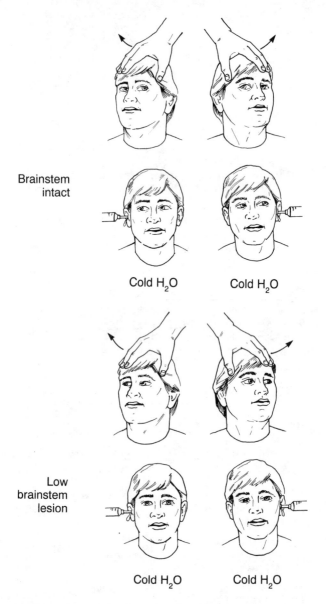

Brainstem
intact

Cold H$_2$O   Cold H$_2$O

Low
brainstem
lesion

Cold H$_2$O   Cold H$_2$O

Figure 7–1. Ocular reflexes and caloric testing in the unconscious patient.

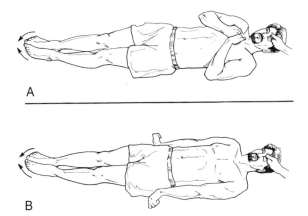

Figure 7–2. *(A)* Decorticate and *(B)* decerebrate posturing in response to a painful stimulus.

Ancillary Tests

Lab tests should include CBC, chemistries (including calcium and magnesium), ABG, ECG, and a CT scan of the head. If meningitis is suspected, a lumbar puncture (LP) should be performed. Timing of the LP is sometimes controversial because there is a theoretic risk of herniation if the ICP is elevated. Some prefer to wait for the CT scan. If you choose to wait, but you think meningitis is a real possibility, draw blood cultures and give antibiotics immediately! You can then do the LP later and at least get a sample for a Gram's stain and immunoelectrophoresis of bacterial antigens. Other CSF tests to send include the cell count (looking for infection or hemorrhage), glucose (low in infection), and protein (elevated in infection or some neurologic diseases), and culture. Toxicologic screens and an ethanol level should be considered, as indicated by the particular circumstances and findings.

Disposition

Comatose patients should be admitted to an ICU, or to the operating room if a neurosurgical emergency is found on the head CT scan. In very rare cases, when a treatable cause is found and the patient recovers rapidly, admission to a floor bed or discharge is possible.

SEIZURES

This section will briefly outline our approach to the actively "seizing" patient without head trauma. Each step, unless otherwise noted, assumes that the seizures are still continuing. Throughout the care of the patient, we assume you will constantly be reassessing the patient's ABCs. Remember to test anticonvulsant levels if the patient has been receiving such therapy, as the most common reason for a seizure is inadequate blood levels of a prescribed anticonvulsant. Pertinent labs in patients with a first-time seizure should include a CBC, electrolytes, calcium, magnesium, glucose, BUN and creatinine, and a head CT scan. The treatment protocol is as follows:

1. Evaluate the ABCs. Look for and treat hypoxia, hypotension, and hypoglycemia.
2. Establish IV access, and give thiamine 100 mg IV.
3. Give lorazepam 0.05 mg/kg (usually 4 mg in an adult) IV over 2 minutes.
4. In 3 to 5 minutes, repeat the same dose of lorazepam.
5. If the seizure is continuing, *or* has responded to lorazepam, give phenytoin 15 to 18 mg/kg (usually 1 g in an adult) IV slowly, *no faster* than 0.5 mg/kg per minute. Monitor very closely for

hypotension; if it occurs, stop the drip until it resolves; then resume at a slower rate.

6. If the seizure continues, give phenobarbital 10 mg/kg IV at 1 mg/kg per minute. This may be repeated up to twice more, to a maximum 30 mg/kg if necessary.

7. By this point, neurologic consultation should be available. If seizures continue, consider clonazepam, paraldehyde, barbiturate coma, lidocaine, a midazolam drip, or general anesthesia with electroencephalographic (EEG) monitoring.

STROKES

A patient who has had a cerebrovascular event usually will present with a focal neurologic deficit, such as aphasia or hemiparesis. Your first priority, as always, is to stabilize the patient (i.e., the ABCs). Some patients will require intubation for altered mental status; all patients with possible stroke should receive oxygen. Ensure that the patient is hemodynamically stable. Begin cardiac monitoring. Look for and treat hypoglycemia. Obtain IV access and order an ECG, as occasionally an MI can present with an embolic stroke from a ventricular thrombus. Once the patient is stabilized, a further diagnostic workup can be carried out. Early noncontrast head CT scanning is mandatory to rule out a hemorrhage.

Strokes generally have one of three etiologies: hemorrhagic, thrombotic, or embolic. *Hemorrhagic stroke* patients generally present with severe headache; such patients often are hypertensive. Vomiting and nuchal rigidity may be present. A preceding headache usually is noted. *Thrombotic stroke* usually is seen in patients with severe carotid atherosclerosis; they often present with a history of several hours or days of progressing symptoms. *Embolic stroke* is the most common type. It usually occurs in inadequately anticoagulated patients who have atrial fibrillation, a recent MI with a mural thrombus, or cardiac ventricular aneurysms. They usually experience sudden onset of an unchanging symptom complex. All patients with stroke should be admitted for monitoring and treatment.

A note on terminology: A *transient ischemic attack* (TIA) is a stroke-like syndrome that lasts less than 24 hours. A *reversible ischemic neurologic deficit* (RIND) lasts more than 24 hours but clears completely. Obviously these diagnoses may be made only in retrospect. In general, a patient who presents with a resolving or resolved neurologic deficit that seems stroke-like should be treated identically to a patient with a persistent deficit.

NONTRAUMATIC HEADACHE

Patients who present to the ED with headache want pain relief. They also may be quite worried that they have a brain tumor, and they will want a CT scan or MRI of their brain. In general, most of them will not need any studies, but certain H&P findings should prompt you to pursue the possibility of serious disease aggressively.

Patients with headache and fever should be assessed extremely carefully for meningitis. Ask about photophobia or vomiting. Look for meningismus. If you suspect meningitis, an LP is mandatory unless the patient has signs of increased ICP (such as papilledema) or focal neurologic deficits. In those cases, draw blood cultures, give antibiotics, and order a head CT scan to rule out a mass lesion before performing the LP.

Any headache patient with new focal neurologic

deficits or confusion, or with a severe sudden-onset headache, should have a head CT performed. (Look for subarachnoid hemorrhage; be aware that these patients need an LP if the CT is negative.) Immunosuppressed patients and those with a history consistent with tumor (a prolonged course of slowly worsening headache, especially worse on awakening) also should have a head CT, as should any patient with chronic headache who has a new type of headache, unless an obviously benign cause is found. Be especially wary if a patient says this is the "worst headache of my life"; usually he or she should be scanned.

Migraine Headache

Migraine is a very common reason for patients with headache to present to the ED. Often the pain is typical of their migraine headaches but worse in intensity and unresponsive to their available home therapies. First ask them what they have received previously in EDs and how well it worked; often this will give you a good idea of what to treat them with. Many general options are available as well. We like to use prochlorperazine (Compazine) 5 to 10 mg IV (in an adult) as a first-line agent, especially for those with nausea accompanying the headache; if that hasn't improved the pain in 20 minutes, we give dihydroergotamine (DHE) 1 mg IV. This drug is a vasoconstrictor and cannot be given to patients with coronary or cerebral vascular disease. Another option is sumatriptan 6 mg SC; this may be repeated once if the first dose doesn't work. Note that this drug is also a vasoconstrictor with the same cautions as DHE. Finally, of course, one can use IM or IV analgesics such as morphine; this usually relieves pain primarily by putting the patient to sleep. Before treating these patients with an opioid analgesic, which may mask subtle neurologic findings, these patients must have a complete history and neurologic examination.

8

CHAPTER

Acute Eye Problems

If a patient has any eye complaints, check his or her visual acuity before examining the rest of the eye, unless there is obvious severe trauma, such as a pencil penetrating the eyeball. Always assess pupillary response and extraocular movements, and look for foreign bodies under both upper and lower lids. The upper eyelid should always be everted over a cotton swab. Slit lamp examination (Fig. 8–1) and fluorescein staining, direct ophthalmoscopy, and ocular pressure measurement complete the eye examination. Topical anesthesia, such as tetracaine or proparacaine eye drops, may assist you in performing the exam. Also consider and look for systemic disorders such as temporal arteritis in the patient with eye pain.

True ophthalmologic emergencies that always require immediate consultation include:

- Acute visual loss
- Chemical burns to the eye
- Penetrating eye injuries
- Acute angle closure glaucoma

THE RED EYE

Most patients with a red and painful eye will have one of the following complaints, which you can sort out rapidly based on the H&P exam:

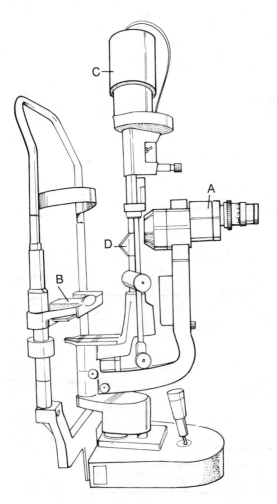

Figure 8–1. The slit lamp: *(A)* stereoscopic micro-scope; *(B)* patient's chin rest; *(C)* light source; *(D)* adjustable slit mechanism.

Vision Decreased

Narrow Angle Glaucoma.   This is a true emergency. These patients have extremely high intraocular pressure. They also have decreased vision, photophobia, eye pain, nausea, and vomiting, and they often complain of seeing halos around lights. The pupil is fixed, and the cornea is often cloudy or "steamy." Ocular pressure will be greater than 20 mm Hg. Obtain an immediate ophthalmologic consultation. Begin treatment with pilocarpine eye drops, beta-blocker eye drops, IV acetazolamide (500 mg), and IV mannitol (1 g/kg).

Uveitis.   This inflammation of the iris, ciliary body, or choroid can be caused by a local infection or an immune response secondary to a systemic disorder (e.g., Crohn's disease), although the cause often is unclear. These patients have eye pain, photophobia, and often decreased vision. The pupil usually is constricted. Ciliary flush (injection of vessels around the corneal limbus) usually is present. Slit-lamp exam may show anterior chamber inflammation ("cells and flare"). These patients should be referred urgently to an ophthalmologist.

Vision Usually Normal

Conjunctivitis.   Usually this presents with ocular discharge and itching, without decrease in vision, and with conjunctival inflammation on exam. These patients can be treated with sulfacetamide or erythromycin topically (available as drops or ointments) for 7 days. Two notable exceptions to this are: 1) *herpetic conjunctivitis*, which also involves the cornea, with dendritic ulcers seen on fluorescein exam, and requires an immediate ophthalmologic consultation and admission; and 2) *gonococcal conjunctivitis*, which usually produces profuse, purulent exudates and requires systemic treatment with penicillin along with topical antibiotics.

Corneal Abrasions. These usually produce pain, itching, or a foreign-body sensation in the eye, without visual compromise. The patient may give a history of mild trauma to the eye. Be sure there is no perforation of the globe. Always look for and remove any foreign bodies. Fluorescein will reveal the extent of the corneal lesion. In the past, these patients often had their eyes patched, but this probably is not necessary for either healing or comfort. Corneal abrasions secondary to use of contact lenses should not be patched. We usually give patients with corneal abrasions antibiotic ointment to apply four times a day to the eye, and we instruct them to return if they are not better in 24 hours. All of these patients should receive tetanus prophylaxis as indicated (see Chapter 15). Table 8–1 summarizes the differential diagnosis of the red eye.

ACUTE VISUAL LOSS

Acute binocular vision loss almost always involves the CNS, specifically problems with the vertebrobasilar circulation. Therefore, in a patient presenting with sudden blindness, your workup should proceed as for a patient with a stroke or TIA (see Chapter 7). Note, though, that some patients with migraine headaches can experience associated visual loss; unless they give this history, however, consider this a diagnosis of exclusion. In all patients with new binocular blindness, ophthalmologic consultation is mandatory.

Monocular visual loss can be due to either eye disorders or CNS problems. Patients who have CNS causes usually present with hemianopsia

Table 8–1. DIFFERENTIAL DIAGNOSIS OF THE RED EYE

History and Clinical Findings	Conjunctivitis	Iritis	Acute Glaucoma	Corneal Infection (Bacterial Ulcer)	Corneal Ulcer
Incidence	Very common	Common	Common	Common	Common
Onset	Insidious	Insidious	Sudden	Slow	Sudden
Vision	Normal	Slightly blurred	Markedly blurred	Usually blurred	Blurred
Pain	None to moderate	Moderate	Severe	Moderate to severe	Severe
Photophobia	None to mild	Severe	Minimal	Variable	Moderate
Nausea and vomiting	None	None	Occasional	None	None
Discharge	Moderate to copious	None	None	Watery	Watery
Ciliary injection	Absent	Present, circumcorneal	Present	Present	Present

(Continued)

Table 8-1. (*Continued*)

History and Clinical Findings	Conjunctivitis	Iritis	Acute Glaucoma	Corneal Infection (Bacterial Ulcer)	Corneal Ulcer
Conjunctival injection	Severe, diffuse	Minimal	Minimal	Moderate	Mild
Cornea	Clear	Clear	Steamy	Hazy	Hazy
Stain with fluorescein	Absent	Absent	Absent	Present	Present
Hypopyon	Absent	Occasional	Absent	Occasional	Absent
Pupil size	Normal	Constricted	Midposition, fixed	Normal	Normal
Intraocular pressure	Normal	Normal	Elevated	Normal	Normal
Pupillary light response	Normal	Poor	None	Normal	Normal

rather than monocular blindness. True monocular vision loss directs you to look for problems at the eye or optic nerve. The specific disorders you are likely to encounter are optic neuritis or neuropathy, retinal detachment, vitreous hemorrhage, and central retinal artery occlusion. In all of these cases, ophthalmologic consultation is mandatory. In some cases, emergency therapy will be required.

Optic Nerve Disease

Most commonly called optic neuritis, optic nerve disease will cause *visual loss and pain* behind the affected eye. About 30% of patients with optic neuritis will develop multiple sclerosis (MS). It is now generally accepted that the standard of care for optic neuritis is admission for IV glucocorticoid therapy to reduce the patient's likelihood of developing MS.

Retinal Detachment

Retinal detachment can occur after trauma or in patients predisposed to retinal hemorrhage, such as diabetics or patients with coagulopathies. Monocular painless loss of vision is accompanied by a "shadow or curtain" sensation coming down over the affected eye. The detachment may not be visualized easily with the direct ophthalmoscope, so if you suspect this diagnosis, call the ophthalmologist. Therapy involves laser "tacking" of the retina.

Vitreous Hemorrhage

Vitreous hemorrhage is most commonly seen in diabetics and in patients with bleeding disorders.

It involves bleeding into the vitreous chamber. You will most likely only see a red haze on funduscopy.

Giant Cell Arteritis

Also known as temporal arteritis, giant cell arteritis typically presents in patients older than 50 and is associated with headache, jaw claudication, visual loss, and a markedly elevated erythrocyte sedimentation rate (ESR). Polymyalgia rheumatica also may be present. A temporal artery may be tender. High-dose oral steroids (such as prednisone, 60 mg per day) must be started to try to prevent visual loss in the other eye.

Central Retinal Artery Occlusion

Central retinal artery occlusion can be caused by cholesterol emboli, thrombotic emboli, or vasculitis. It is much more common in the elderly, who have a much higher incidence of carotid atherosclerotic disease. The retina will appear pale, with the macula looking like a cherry-red spot in the whitish-yellow background. You may see blood stains ("box-carring"), or even the embolus itself. Begin treatment immediately; your goal is to lower the intraocular pressure so as to force the embolus more peripherally and perhaps preserve retinal tissue.

1. Give mannitol 1 g/kg IV and acetazolamide 500 mg IV to reduce production of aqueous humor.
2. Apply beta-blockers or pilocarpine eye drops.
3. "Ballot" the eye by applying intermittent pressure to the eyeball for 15 seconds out of every minute ("CPR of the eyeball").
4. Obtain an ophthalmologic consultation immediately to maximize the chances of vision salvage.

Central retinal *vein* occlusion occurs in the same age group and also causes monocular painless visual loss. Funduscopic examination reveals a blood-streaked retina. Even though no specific treatment exists, immediate consultation also is required.

OTHER EYE EMERGENCIES

Penetrating Eye Injuries

Although sometimes obvious, penetrating eye injuries may not always be apparent, especially when they involve the posterior part of the eye. A teardrop-shaped pupil suggests eye penetration with herniation of the iris through the wound. Visual acuity usually is reduced and the globe is soft. The eye should be protected with a rigid eye shield. The base of a plastic or styrofoam cup can be used to protect the eye from protrusion in the absence of a metal shield. The patient also should receive IV antibiotics (cefazolin 1 g and gentamicin 1.5 mg/kg) while waiting to see the ophthalmologist.

Chemical Burns of the Eyes

Chemical (especially alkali) burns, which cause liquefaction necrosis, can result in major tissue destruction. Immediate irrigation with 1 to 2 liters NS should be performed. Larger volumes of irrigant may be required to return the pH in the eye to normal. Irrigation can be facilitated by using a topical anesthetic to relieve the pain and any blepharospasm. It is helpful to check the pH of the eye 5 minutes after irrigation to ensure that a physiologic pH has been attained.

9

CHAPTER

Low Back Pain

Most people suffer from back pain sometime in their life, and it is considered one of the most common presentations to the ED. Back injuries are the single most costly health problem for working America.

Although it has many causes, low back pain (LBP) usually is the result of benign conditions and will respond to conservative treatment such as bed rest, NSAIDs, local heat, and muscle relaxants. Your job is to identify those patients with serious, life-threatening, underlying diseases (such as a leaking or ruptured abdominal aortic aneurysm or an aortic dissection). You must also recognize spinal cord compression and disorders that impair neurologic function, and decide who needs urgent workup, admission, or immediate consultation. Be especially diligent at the extremes of age. Children rarely complain of LBP, so assume it has a serious cause, and the elderly often have serious underlying conditions. Rather than reviewing the extensive list of differential diagnoses, this chapter will present a practical approach to patients with LBP.

HISTORY

The following information should be obtained from all patients:

- Is there any history of recent or remote injury?
- What were the circumstances of onset of pain? Has there been any recent unusual physical exertion or heavy lifting?
- Is the pain acute or chronic?
- Is there any associated chest pain, abdominal pain, pelvic pain, or difficulty breathing?
- Does the pain radiate to the groin or leg?
- Is the pain in the leg exacerbated by sneezing, coughing, or defecating?
- If the pain radiates to the leg, is there pain below the knee? (Radiation of pain below the knee is more specific for true sciatica.)
- Is there a history of symptoms suggestive of malignant disease? (This increases the likelihood of spinal metastases.)
- Have there been any changes in bowel or bladder function?
- Is there any numbness or weakness in the legs?
- Has there been any burning sensation on urination? Has the patient been urinating more frequently than usual?
- Is there a history of fever or chills? (This may suggest an infectious process.)
- Is the patient taking steroids or immunosuppressants? (Think of osteoporosis and infections.)
- Is the patient an IV drug abuser? (This increases the chances of an epidural abscess.)
- Is the patient taking oral anticoagulants? (Consider retroperitoneal bleeding.)
- Has the patient received any therapy for the pain?

PHYSICAL EXAMINATION

Observe the patient before he or she realizes that you have begun your assessment. Often the posture and facial expression will change dramatically as soon as you enter the room. If possible have the patient stand up; note how easy it is for him or her to get up. Look at the patient's back. Are there any obvious deformities (scoliosis or kyphosis)? Is there evidence of trauma? Palpate the length of the spinal column, paravertebral musculature, buttocks, and flanks for areas of tenderness or muscle spasm. Have the patient point to the area of maximal discomfort. Have the patient stand and test to see how far forward he or she can bend at the waist. An increase in pain may suggest a disk problem. Assessing range of motion is, however, very subjective and may not always be helpful. Ask the patient to walk on heels (this tests foot dorsiflexion) and toes (this tests foot plantar flexion). Next have the patient sit on the edge of the examining table to assess for deep tendon reflexes (if you don't have a reflex hammer, you can use the head of your stethoscope). Test the ankle (S_1) and knee (L_3, L_4) reflexes in both legs. Many patients will not have good reflexes. Distracting the patient can help elicit deep tendon reflexes. While still sitting, listen for breath sounds and auscultate the heart. (In rare cases, a pneumothorax may present as sudden onset of sharp pleuritic back pain.)

Have the patient lie supine and examine the abdomen for a pulsating mass (aortic aneurysm), hepatomegaly, or discrete masses (may suggest malignancy). Listen for abdominal or flank bruits. Check for femoral and pedal pulses. Women will require a full pelvic examination unless the cause of their back pain is readily apparent. Pay particular attention to the presence of fever, lymphadenopathy, or any needle "track marks."

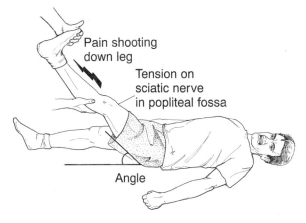

Figure 9–1. Straight-leg raising eliciting pain, which radiates down the leg. The pain is exacerbated by dorsiflexing the foot and putting tension on the sciatic nerve in the popliteal fossa.

Straight leg raising (SLR) tests for true sciatica, indicating a radicular origin of the pain. Passively flex the outstretched legs at the hip and see if, and at what level (expressed as degrees), pain shoots down the leg (Fig. 9–1). Back pain is not considered a positive finding. Helpful hints: Dorsiflexion of the foot will increase true sciatica, whereas flexion at the knee will decrease the pain elicited during SLR. Increased pain on raising the contralateral leg (crossed SLR) is even more specific for a radicular origin of the pain.

It may be difficult to determine whether there is a functional, nonorganic component of the patient's LBP. (Be aware, also, that most *chronic* LBP has a psychologic component.) Helpful hints that one is dealing with a patient with a functional disorder include the following:

- Applying pressure to the top of the head is reported to increase LBP (it should not).

- Hip or shoulder rotation is reported to increase LBP (it should not).
- Compare SLR lying and sitting.
- Patient is overreacting.

Spinal Cord Syndromes

Disease processes involving the spinal cord and its elements usually present as one of two symptom complexes:

1. **Radiculopathy** is due to pressure on spinal roots. Usually only one or a few segmental levels are involved, and the patient presents with sharp segmental pain and loss of sensation and motor weakness at the corresponding level. If the muscle is involved in a deep tendon reflex arc, the reflex will be weak or absent.
2. **Myelopathy** is secondary to pressure on the spinal cord itself. The patient presents with partial or total loss of sensory and motor function below the level of the lesion.

THE NEUROLOGIC EXAMINATION

It is helpful to assess each of the three spinal cord sections separately:

1. **The anterior cord** is assessed by testing the gross motor function of various muscle groups and cord levels.
2. **The lateral cord** is assessed by testing for pinprick sensation or two-point discrimination.
3. **The posterior cord** is assessed by testing proprioception (sense of positioning), vibration sensation, or both. Have patients close their eyes and indicate whether you are pointing their big toe downwards or upwards.

Table 9–1 will help you determine the level of the spinal cord lesion based on clinical findings.

Since most neurologic deficits result from disc herniation and most herniations are at the level of L4–5 or L5–S1, particular emphasis should be placed on testing toe dorsiflexion and plantar flexion, sensation between the first and second toes and on the undersurface of the foot, and the presence or absence of an ankle jerk.

A rectal exam is always a good idea, but especially in the presence of:

- Any neurologic deficit
- Symptoms of bowel or bladder dysfunction
- A recent change in bowel habits or rectal bleeding
- An elderly man in whom prostatic cancer is likely

Detailed assessment for saddle anesthesia (the perineal region) should be performed whenever a rectal exam is done. A rough assessment for saddle anesthesia can be made by pinching the patient's

Table 9–1. DETERMINING THE LEVEL OF SPINAL CORD INVOLVEMENT

Level of Lesion	Level of Sensory Loss	Motor Deficit	Lost Reflex
L1	Groin crease	Hip flexion	—
L2, L3	Medial thigh	Hip adduction	—
L4	Knee	Hip abduction	Patellar
L5	Lateral calf, first toe webspace	Foot and big toe dorsiflexion	—
S1	Lateral foot	Foot and big toe plantar flexion	Achilles
S2–S4	Perianal region	Rectal sphincter tone	—

buttocks. (Explain to the patient why you are doing this!)

ANCILLARY TESTS

In most patients, a detailed H&P exam are enough to rule out serious pathology. Other tests may be indicated for some patients:

X-rays of the lumbosacral spine are indicated in the following circumstances:

- Recent significant trauma
- Evidence of malignant disease anywhere in the body
- Age extremes (<18 years and >50 years old)
- Unresolved back pain > 10 days
- Prior to referral to a specialist
- Fever, weight loss, adenopathy, or signs of systemic illness
- History of IV drug abuse or alcohol abuse
- History of tuberculosis (Pott's disease)
- Neurologic deficits
- Intended litigation or compensation

A significantly elevated *ESR* suggests metastatic disease, infectious disease, or inflammatory disease.

If you suspect renal calculi or infection, perform a dipstick or full *urinalysis*.

In patients older than 50 with lower flank or back pain, especially if they are hypotensive, consider performing an immediate bedside *ultrasound* to exclude an abdominal aortic aneurysm.

ACUTE SPINAL CORD COMPRESSION

The acute onset of spinal cord compression is a medical emergency requiring urgent surgical decompression or radiation therapy.

Patients with spinal cord compression usually present with loss of sensation and motor function below the level of compression, with some degree of bowel and/or bladder dysfunction. The causes of acute cord compression include:

- **Tumors:** primary or secondary (e.g., lung, breast, prostate, lymphoma, multiple myeloma)
- **Infections:** epidural abscess
- **Trauma:** dislocation of the vertebra or vertebral body collapse
- **Disc injury:** ruptured intervertebral disc or severe central herniation or compression
- **Hematoma:** spontaneous or traumatic

Often there is segmental involvement of spinal roots at the level of the lesion, and the patient presents with unilateral or bilateral pain radiating in a dermatomal pattern or with radicular paresthesias. All patients with acute spinal cord compression need immediate admission and a workup that includes plain films of the spine (look for vertebral body collapse, bony erosions, or paraspinal soft tissue masses) and MRI (or CT scanning with metrizamide myelography).

All patients should be immobilized adequately before you proceed with any diagnostic or therapeutic measures. For patients with traumatic spinal cord injuries, give an IV bolus of methylprednisolone 30 mg/kg within 8 hours of injury, followed by 5.4 mg/kg per hour over the next 23 hours.

DISPOSITION

Most patients with LBP, even in the presence of stable isolated neurologic deficits, can be sent home safely. Indications for admission include:

- Acute spinal cord compression
- Serious underlying diseases (e.g., abdominal or thoracic aneurysm)
- Spinal cord infections
- Intractable pain (rarely the sole indication)
- Multiple nerve root involvement
- Progressive or severe neurologic impairment
- Unstable fractures, traumatic dislocations or subluxation
- Acute spinal trauma and neurologic deficits

MANAGEMENT

The following are general recommendations for outpatient management of patients with acute LBP:

1. **Strict bed rest:** Patients are instructed to lie in whatever position is comfortable, with only bathroom privileges are allowed at home. More than 48 to 72 hours of bed rest has not been found to be more beneficial than a shorter period of bed rest.
2. **Anti-inflammatory medications:** Most causes of LBP have an inflammatory component in their course. Aspirin or NSAIDs may be effective. The choice of a specific agent should be individualized. Always make sure that the patient does not have a history of a bleeding ulcer or allergy to the particular medicine chosen. These medications can irritate the stomach and should be given with foods or antacids.

3. **Muscle relaxants:** Their use is controversial. In the presence of significant paravertebral muscle spasm, they may help break the pain-spasm-pain cycle. Also, their sedative effect helps ensure strict bed rest. Warn patients about driving and operating dangerous machinery while taking these medications. Diazepam (2 to 5 mg PO tid) probably is the most effective muscle relaxant. Alternatives include cyclobenzaprine (10 mg PO tid) or methocarbamol (1500 mg PO tid).
4. **Analgesics:** Acetaminophen with codeine or hydrocodone can be added every 4 to 6 hours if necessary.
5. **Local measures:** Whether it is better to apply heat or cold to the painful area is controversial. Whatever makes the patient feel better should be offered.

PROGNOSIS

Within 6 weeks, 90% of episodes of acute LBP will respond to treatment or resolve spontaneously. Although approximately 5% of patients will require admission, only 1% require surgery. Patients should be instructed to return to the ED if they develop any bladder or bowel dysfunction or progressive muscle weakness in the legs.

Remember never to assume malingering or that nothing is wrong. The patient's pain is always real to the patient.

10

Poisonings and Principles of Toxicology

Toxicology is one of the most challenging aspects of emergency medicine. Like an astute detective, you must use all of your senses (except for taste) to gather information from the patient, family, friends, and EMS personnel to help detect the poison ingested by the patient. The H&P and initial laboratory results will supply you with the essential pieces required to help solve the poisoning puzzle.

Many health care workers are "turned off" by the intoxicated or suicidal patient. Don't be judgmental. Instead, meet the challenge the patient presents, and you will be rewarded.

RECOGNIZING POISONINGS

The most important factor in determining the outcome in acute poisonings is early recognition that one is in fact dealing with a toxicologic problem. Generally, it is wise to consider a poisoning in all patients presenting to the ED. In the following situations, particularly, you should ask yourself whether the patient's condition is secondary to an acute or chronic poisoning:

- An altered mental status
- Abnormal vital signs not readily explained by other underlying pathology
- Anion gap metabolic acidosis
- A significant osmolar gap
- A patient who is depressed or suicidal
- A known history of prior overdose
- Children between ages 1 to 5 years and 11 to 18 years
- When the patient or family states that the patient swallowed pills
- When EMS personnel find empty pill containers at the scene of injury
- Classic signs and symptoms of a toxidrome
- Psychiatric patients on medications
- Elderly patients on cardiac medications
- Unexplained illness after ingesting food, drink, or medication
- Multiple individuals whose illnesses all began at the same time

It is important to remember that in cases of poisoning, the historic information obtained from bystanders may be inaccurate or even misleading. Always maintain a high index of suspicion.

Patients with poisonings may present with no symptoms at all. When their toxicity is delayed, you must focus on preventing drug absorption and monitoring for evidence of toxicity. IV access, continuous cardiac monitoring, and frequent reevaluations are necessary in all patients with a potential poisoning.

In many situations, laboratory confirmation of a specific poison is not available in the ED. Initiation of both nonspecific and specific therapy must be based on your clinical judgment, with the urgency dictated by the gravity of the patient's condition.

Regional poison control centers can provide an invaluable source of information.

INITIAL ASSESSMENT

All poisoning patients require a rapid assessment of their ABCs; resuscitation and stabilization often is begun before any information is available. Don't let EMS personnel leave before you obtain as much information as possible concerning a potential overdose. If the EMS personnel are unsure, send them back to the scene, if possible, to collect any evidence. Other sources of information include friends, pharmacists, or the patient's physicians. The following are important questions to ask:

- What were the patient's vital signs and initial mental status at the scene?
- What therapy was given en route to the hospital?
- Was there any evidence of intoxication?
- Were any pill containers found?
- What medications were found? (Find out the names, strengths, and original and present number of pills.) Was there any possibility of exposure to environmental toxins?
- What is the patient's occupation?
- Where does the patient work?
- When did the overdose occur?
- When was the patient last seen?

Physical Examination

The physical exam assumes the utmost importance because it often elicits vital clues to the nature of the poisoning. Perform a detailed physical exam with particular emphasis on vital signs, neurologic exam, skin, and diagnostic odors. A detailed list of effects of specific toxins on the various organ systems is presented in Appendix B. We do not find these exhaustive lists helpful; instead a combination of signs and symptoms produced by a toxin or a category of toxins may be useful.

TOXIDROMES

Once you suspect a poisoning, try to determine whether the pattern of signs and symptoms fits into any particular toxidrome (toxic syndrome). The more common toxidromes are:

- Anticholinergics
- Cholinergics
- Sympathomimetics
- Opioids
- Withdrawal of substances of abuse
- Anion gap metabolic acidosis

Anticholinergics

Clinical Manifestations: Patients may present with tachycardia, tachypnea, hypertension, hyperthermia, convulsions, hallucinations, mydriasis, flushed skin, hypoactive bowel sounds, thirst, and/or urinary retention. To help you remember the signs of anticholinergic overdose think of "Alice in Wonderland":

- Mad as a hatter
- Hot as a hare
- Blind as a bat
- Dry as a bone
- Red as a beet

Examples. Antihistamines, antispasmodic gastrointestinal preparations, antiparkinsonian drugs, atropine, benztropine, cyclic antidepressants, phenothiazines, mydriatic ophthalmic agents, over-the-counter sleep medications (always ask about the use of over-the-counter medications), and jimson weed.

Cholinergics

Clinical Manifestations. The mnemonic **DUMBBELSS** will help you remember the signs of cholingeric overdose:

D = defecation
U = urination
M = miosis
B = bradycardia
B = bronchospasm
E = emesis
L = lacrimation
S = secretions
S = seizures

Examples. Organophosphate insecticides, carbamate insecticides, edrophonium, some toxic mushrooms, pilocarpine, betel nut.

Sympathomimetics

Clinical Manifestations. Patients may present with CNS excitation, convulsions, hypertension, tachycardia, mydriasis, tremors, and/or diaphoresis. *This toxidrome is very similar to the anticholinergic toxidrome;* the use of sympathomimetics can be assumed, however, when active bowel sounds and diaphoresis are present.

Examples. Cocaine, amphetamines, caffeine, theophylline, phencyclidine (**PCP**), lysergic acid diethylamide (LSD), phenylpropanolamine (a common component of diet pills and decongestants).

Opioids

Clinical Manifestations. Classically, patients present with a clinical triad of hypoventilation, CNS depression, and miosis (miosis is absent, however, with meperidine and diphenoxylate). Hypotension also is common. Emergent treatment with naloxone rarely is indicated unless respiratory compromise is present or you are unsure of the diagnosis. Consider applying physical restraints before administering an antagonist, which can result in severe agitation.

Examples. Heroin, morphine, codeine, propoxyphene, pentazocine, diphenoxylate, meperidine.

Withdrawal of Substances of Abuse

Clinical Manifestations. Patients may present with tachycardia, diarrhea, vomiting, mydriasis, gooseflesh, lacrimation, cramps, yawning, agitation, and/or seizures.

Examples. Opioids, alcohol, barbiturates, chloral hydrate.

INITIAL MANAGEMENT

Always start by assessing the patient's ABCs. Patients who are lethargic or unresponsive often will need to be intubated to protect their airway. All patients with an altered mental status should receive the following treatment:

1. 100% **O₂** via a non-rebreather mask.
2. **Thiamine** 100 mg IV (should be given before glucose).
3. **Glucose** should be checked with a glucose oxidase indicator strip (Dextrostix, Ames Co., Elkhart, IN). If a glucose level is not immediately available or if it is < 60 to 80 mg/dL, give 50 mL $D_{50}W$ IV push (2 to 4 mL D_{25}W/kg in children).
4. **Naloxone** 2 mg IV (0.1 mg/kg up to 2 mg in children). You may consider giving up to 20 mg IV, especially in the setting of propoxyphene, meperidine, or oxycodone overdose.

NONSPECIFIC THERAPY

The following treatment guidelines are aimed at decreasing the absorption and enhancing the elimination of potential toxins.

Gastric Decontamination

Activated Charcoal

Activated charcoal is the most effective decontaminant. It acts by adsorbing toxin present in the gastrointestinal tract. Even when gastric lavage is indicated, activated charcoal should be administered via the orotracheal tube before lavage. Adults should receive 50 to 100 g PO (give children 1 to 2 g/kg). Use the mnemonic **CHARCOAL** to remember the substances that are *not* adsorbed by activated charcoal:

C = caustics and corrosives
H = heavy metals

A = alcohols and glycols
R = rapidly absorbed substances
C = cyanide
O = other insoluble drugs
A = aliphatic hydrocarbons
L = laxatives

Other contraindications of the use of activated charcoal include absent bowel sounds or other signs of intestinal obstruction or perforation.

Gastric Lavage

Gastric lavage usually is effective only if performed within 30 to 60 minutes of toxic ingestion (it still may be effective even if given later in intoxications with substances that slow down gastrointestinal motility, such as anticholinergics). Gastric lavage has been shown to be less effective than activated charcoal. It is indicated in toxic ingestions of substances not absorbed by activated charcoal or in unstable patients in whom intubation is indicated. The patient should be placed in the left lateral position with the head lower than the hips. Use a large orogastric tube (36F to 40F in adults and 16F to 28F in children). Lavage never should be performed in patients with actual or potential mental obtundation or seizures without prior protection of the airway with a cuffed endotracheal tube. (Cuffed tubes are not appropriate in children younger than 6 years.) Lavage with aliquots of 250 mL NS (50 to 100 mL in children) until gastrointestinal contents are clear. Attach a 60-mL syringe (whose plunger has been removed) to the tube, and pour NS directly into the syringe; then drain using gravity or low suction (Fig. 10–1). An oral airway may be placed between the teeth to prevent biting down on the tube should the patient awaken or seize. Before removal, pinch off the tube to avoid dripping fluid down into the airway. *Absolute contraindications to gastric lavage include:*

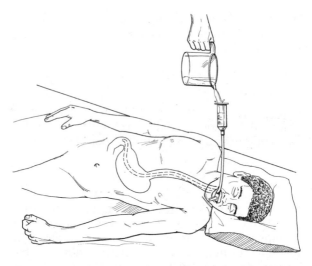

Figure 10–1. Gastic lavage: the patient is placed in the left lateral position with the head down.

- Caustic ingestions
- Intestinal obstruction
- Intestinal perforation
- Age less than 9 months old

Ipecac

Although possibly useful in the home setting, ipecac is rarely indicated in the ED. Ipecac is given to patients with recent (within 30 minutes) mushroom or unknown plant ingestions in which gastric lavage would be ineffective. Adults should receive 30 to 60 mL PO; children > 15 months, 15 mL PO; and children < 15 months, 10 mL PO. Avoid giving ipecac to any patient with the potential for rapid deterioration of mental status (e.g., those who have ingested cyclic antidepressants) or development of seizures. Other contraindications include ingestion of corrosives, caustics, petroleum distillates, or foreign bodies; loss of the gag reflex; unstable patients; age less than 6 months; and when the patient has already vomited.

Cathartics

Many cathartics are available, but magnesium citrate is the most useful because of its palatability. (Avoid it if the patient is in renal failure because of the risk of hypermagnesemia.) Adults should receive 30 g PO (300 mL of 10% solution). Sorbitol is an alternate cathartic (give adults 40 mL of 70%). In acetaminophen poisoning, saline sulfate (15 to 30 g PO) is preferred because it can enhance the sulfate metabolic pathway and provide hepatic protection. Cathartics are contraindicated in gastrointestinal bleeding or ileus and should be avoided in children younger than 2 years old.

Enhanced Elimination

Alkalinization of the urine is useful in eliminating weak acids such as salicylates and barbiturates. This is achieved with IV boluses of sodium bicarbonate 8.5% to maintain a urinary pH of 7.5 to 8.0.

Early dialysis may be required in the following poisonings: methyl alcohol, ethylene glycol, *Amanita phalloides* (a poisonous mushroom), aspirin, and lithium. Note that dialysis is most effective with water-soluble agents that have a low volume of distribution (<1 L/kg), poor protein binding (<50%), and low molecular weights (usually <600 d). Charcoal hemoperfusion may be indicated in theophylline overdose. Whole bowel irrigation has been shown to be useful in severe iron overdoses.

ANCILLARY TESTS IN ACUTE POISONINGS

Once you suspect an intoxication, the following labs should be ordered:

1. **Chem 7** (electrolytes, bicarbonate, glucose, BUN, creatinine): This allows you to calculate the anion gap $(Na - [HCO_3 + Cl])$, which helps sort out the various causes of metabolic acidosis (normally $= 10 \pm 2$). The following is a list of common causes of an anion gap metabolic acidosis (use the mnemonic **MUDPILES**):

   M = methanol
   U = uremia
   D = diabetic ketoacidosis
   P = propylene glycol, paraldehyde, phenformin
   I = iron, isoniazide, inhalants (CO, CN, H_2S)
   L = lactic acidosis (seizure, shock, hypoxia)
   E = ethylene glycol, ethanol
   S = salicylates, solvents (toluene).

   A low anion gap suggests the presence of bromides, lithium, or abnormal cationic proteins.

2. **Analysis of ABGs** allows rapid assessment of the oxygenation status and the acid-base balance. Respiratory alkalosis can be an early manifestation of salicylate overdose. The differential diagnosis of acid-base abnormalities is presented in Chapter 2. Carboxyhemoglobin levels should be assessed rapidly if CO poisoning is suspected.

3. **Serum osmolarity:** Calculate the osmolar gap by subtracting the calculated osmolarity from the measured osmolarity. The calculated osmolarity should equal:

$$2 \times Na + \frac{glucose}{18} + \frac{BUN}{2.8} + \frac{Alcohol}{MW \div 10}$$

(Where *MW* = molecular weight of the alcohol.)

Alcohols are the most common cause of an increased osmolar gap. Blood levels of the various alcohols can be estimated from the osmolar gap if their molecular weights are known (ethanol = 46; methanol = 32; ethylene glycol = 62; isopropanol = 60). Other causes of an osmolar gap include isoniazide, mannitol, and trichloroethane. Note, however, that measurements of osmolarity are not always accurate or helpful because of frequent laboratory error.

4. **Acetaminophen level:** Acetaminophen is the most commonly ingested toxin and frequently is a component of a combined overdose. Because there is a known antidote, it is cost-effective to include an acetaminophen level in the "tox labs." Acetaminophen levels should be obtained 4 hours after the ingestion. If the time of ingestion is unknown, it is useful to draw two blood levels at least 1 hour apart and to look for a trend in the levels.

5. **Salicylate level:** This, too, is a common primary or co-ingestant. Levels should be determined 6 hours after ingestion. A level > 30 mg/dL is considered toxic. Treatment never should be delayed if the patient is already symptomatic. The Done nomogram, although widely cited, is not always reliable.

6. **Plain abdominal films** may be helpful if you suspect the ingestion of a radiopaque material (use the mnemonic **CHIPES**):

   C = chloral hydrate, cocaine condoms, calcium, chlorinated hydrocarbons

   H = heavy metals (e.g., arsenic, lead)

   I = iron, iodides

   P = phenothiazines, potassium, Pepto-Bismol, Play-Doh

   E = enteric coated tablets

   S = slow-release capsules, solvents

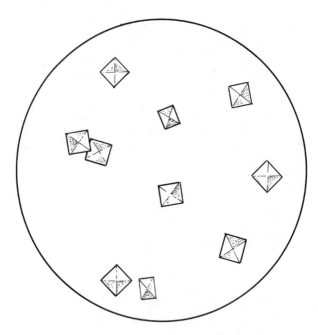

Figure 10–2. Calcium oxalate stones in the urine of a patient with ethylene glycol poisoning.

7. **Specific quantitative laboratory analysis** on an emergent basis should be obtained for the following agents: methanol, ethylene glycol, isopropyl alcohol, iron, theophylline, lithium, CO, digoxin, phenytoin, phenobarbital, and carbamazepine.

8. **Urinalysis:** Microscopic observation of rhomboid or needle-shaped calcium oxalate stones suggests ethylene glycol poisoning (Fig. 10–2). Observe the urine under a Wood's lamp. Fluorescence suggests the presence of antifreeze, a common source of ethlyene glycol (also look for fluorescence around the patient's mouth). If on adding several drops of 10% FeCl, the urine

turns purple, suspect salicylate or phenothiazine poisoning. If the color blanches on adding 20% sulfuric acid, phenothiazines are more likely.

SPECIFIC POISONINGS

Although a detailed review of the clinical manifestations of all toxic substances is not possible here, we will highlight a few of the more common or more lethal substances not already mentioned in the above toxidromes, as well as their specific antidotes when appropriate.

Acetaminophen

Clinical Manifestations. The most common presentation is an asymptomatic patient. Initially there may be nausea, vomiting, and diaphoresis lasting several hours, followed by an asymptomatic phase for 1 to 2 days. Signs of liver dysfunction may be apparent by 48 hours. Occasionally renal impairment may develop. The Rumack-Matthew nomogram (Fig. 10–3) is useful in predicting the probability of hepatic injury based on acetaminophen levels (high-carbohydrate meals or anticholinergics can slow the absorption). (Recently, an extended-release form of acetaminophen has been introduced; the present nomogram may be inappropriate for this agent.) Ingestion of >7.5 g in an adult (>140 mg/kg in children) usually results in toxic acetaminophen levels. Recently, hepatoxicity has been described in fasting patients who ingested as little as 4 to 10 g. In cases of chronic alcoholism and co-ingestion of anticonvulsants, the toxic dose is 50% lower because of the induction of hepatic microsomal oxidases.

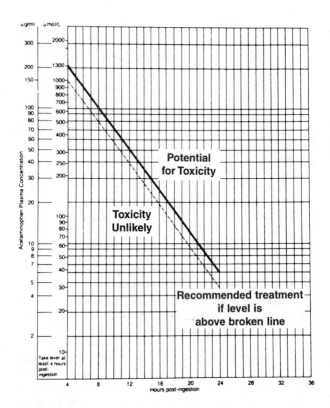

Figure 10–3. The Rumack-Matthew nomogram for acetaminophen overdose. (Reproduced by permission of Pediatrics, Vol. 55, p. 873, copyright 1975.)

Treatment. *N*-acetylcysteine should be given to all patients with toxic acetaminophen levels and estimated ingestions >7.5 g (140 mg/kg in children). An acetaminophen level >5 μg/mL at 24 hours or more postingestion is toxic and might be an indication for acelytcysteine. A loading dose of acetylcysteine 140 mg/kg PO should be followed by 17 maintenance doses of 70 mg/kg PO every 4 hours. Acetylcysteine is <u>most effective if given</u>

within 12 hours of ingestion. It probably is not necessary to increase the dose of acetylcysteine when activated charcoal is administered. If possible, however, try to separate the administration of activated charcoal and acetylcysteine by 1 to 2 hours. Because of its offensive odor, acetylcysteine is not very palatable; dilution of acetylcysteine in chilled fruit juice or tomato juice enhances palatability. If the patient still cannot tolerate the acetylcysteine, administer metaclopramide 10 mg IV or administer acetylcysteine via a nasogastric or nasoduodenal tube. An experimental form of IV acetylcysteine may be available through a poison control center.

Salicylates

Clinical Manifestations. Patients with acute toxicity usually present with vomiting, dehydration, abdominal pain, hyperventilation, diaphoresis, tinnitus, hyperthemia, seizures, bleeding (if severe overdose), and/or a mixed respiratory alkalosis and metabolic acidosis. Pulmonary edema is an uncommon complication. In contrast, chronic toxicity is manifested by alteration in mentation and a mixed acid-base disturbance without gastrointestinal complaints. Adult respiratory distress syndrome (ARDS) is fairly common in cases of chronic toxicity. Chronic toxicity is commonly misdiagnosed and should be suspected especially in the elderly with altered mentation and a mixed acid-base disturbance. Because there is a large volume of distribution in cases of chronic toxicity, salicylate levels do not accurately reflect the degree of toxicity.

Treatment. Correction of dehydration with fluid challenges as well as correction of electrolyte and glucose imbalances may be required. Avoid overhydration, however, which can exacerbate pulmonary or cerebral edema. The arterial pH should be kept > 7.40 to decrease the level of un-ionized salicylates, and the urine should be alkalinized (pH = 7.5 to 8.0) to enhance the urinary excretion of salicylate. Frequent IV boluses of sodium bicarbonate 1 to 2 mEq/kg may be required. Hemodialysis is indicated in the comatose or unstable patient not responding to other measures, in patients with renal failure, and in patients with ARDS with a persistently elevated salicylate level.

Tricyclic Antidepressants

Clinical Manifestations. Tricyclic antidepressants (TCAs) have a quinidine-like effect on the myocardial conducting system, a direct myocardial depressant effect, and an anticholinergic effect. Cardiac dysrhythmias, early tachycardia, hypotension, lengthening of the QRS interval (>0.10 seconds), a rightward shift of the terminal portion of the QRS complex, dystonic movements, convulsions, and coma, as well as other anticholinergic effects, may be present.

Treatment. Alkalinization of the blood (arterial pH = 7.50–7.55) with hyperventilation or frequent IV boluses of sodium bicarbonate 2 mEq/kg enhances mobilization of TCAs from the tissues, while the sodium can reverse the sodium-channel block induced by TCAs. A bicarbonate drip may be necessary. Concomitant hyperventilation and administration of sodium bicarbonate can cause excessive alkalemia and should be avoided. Seizures should be treated with benzodiazepines, phenytoin, or phenobarbital (for details, see Chapter 4). Arrhythmias should be treated with standard measures, but type Ia antiarrhythmics should be avoided.

Theophylline

Clinical Manifestations. Patients present with gastrointestinal irritation, agitation, disorientation, hallucinations, convulsions, cardiac dysrhythmias, hypokalemia, and/or hyperglycemia. Toxicity usually is noted with theophylline levels > 25 to 30 mg/dL. Chronic toxicity manifests at lower levels and does not cause significant gastrointestinal or electrolyte disturbances.

Treatment. Because of its predominantly hepatobiliary enteric circulation, repeated doses of activated charcoal 0.5 g/kg every 2 to 4 hours enhances the elimination of theophylline (gastric dialysis). Seizures and arrhythmias should be managed as usual. Hemodialysis or charcoal hemoperfusion is indicated for severe toxicity or theophylline levels > 100 mg/dL in acute ingestions and > 40 to 60 mg/dL in chronic overdose.

Digoxin

Clinical Manifestations. Patients may present with visual disturbances (seeing yellow-green halos), delirium, gastrointestinal irritation, atrioventricular conduction blocks, ventricular dysrhythmias, and/or hyperkalemia with normal renal function (in acute intoxications). Chronic toxicity is more common in elderly patients with cardiac disease, in whom the serum potassium is either normal or decreased. Ventricular dysrhythmias are more common in chronic toxicity, which can mimic more benign illnesses such as a viral syndrome.

Treatment. Atropine and pacemakers are used for bradyarrhythmias, whereas phenytoin and lidocaine sometimes are effective for ventricular tachyarrhythmias. Digoxin-specific Fab fragments (Digibind, Burroughs Wellcome, Research Triangle Park, NC) are required in the following instances:

- Resistant ventricular arrhythmias or brady-arrhythmias
- Hyperkalemia > 5.5 mEq/L
- A digoxin level > 10 ng/mL at least 6 hours after ingestion

If the exact dose of ingested digoxin is unknown, start by giving 10 ampules of Digibind. Administration of calcium for hyperkalemia should be avoided in cases of digoxin toxicity.

Iron

Clinical Manifestations. Initially, there may be bloody vomitus or diarrhea, leukocytosis, hyperglycemia, an anion gap metabolic acidosis, and/or hypotension. The patient may have a latent asymptomatic phase lasting several hours. This may be followed by hepatic damage, shock, convulsions, or coma. Gastrointestinal obstruction can occur weeks to months later because of strictures.

Treatment. Deferoxamine 15 mg/kg per hour IV should be given until the urine clears. Indications include:

- Ingestion of > 30 mg/kg elemental iron
- Symptomatic patients (regardless of the iron level)
- A serum iron level > 500 µg/dL
- A positive deferoxamine challenge test (give 50 mg/kg IM and see if the urine turns *vin rose* in color)

Note that a patient may have toxic levels of iron even if the level is less than the total iron-binding capacity. Leukocytosis and hyperglycemia suggest more severe toxicity.

Carbon Monoxide

Clinical Manifestations. Signs and symptoms of CO poisoning often appear simultaneously among several members of the same household. Dyspnea, headache, confusion, tachycardia, tachypnea, syncope, seizures, coma, and retinal hemorrhages are common. The venous blood is bright red, resulting in the classical cherry-red appearance of patients. The ABGs are characterized by a metabolic lactic acidosis and initially a normal PaO_2.

Treatment. 100% O_2 should be given by a tight-fitting mask. This will decrease the half life of CO from 5 hours to 90 minutes. Hyperbaric O_2 further decreases the half life of CO to 20 minutes. Indications for hyperbaric O_2 at 3 atm include:

- COHb>25% to 30%
- COHb>15% in children, in patients with significant heart disease, and in symptomatic pregnant patients
- Acute ECG changes
- CNS symptoms (including a *history* of loss of consciousness)
- Severe metabolic acidosis
- Combined CO and cyanide toxicity.

Cyanide

Clinical Manifestations. Patients may present with an odor of bitter almonds on their breath, bradycardia, seizures, coma, and rapid death. The venous blood is bright red, and ABGs indicate metabolic lactic acidosis and initially a normal PaO_2. Cyanide poisoning should be suspected in the comatose, acidotic patient after smoke inhalation, especially in the presence of low CO levels.

Treatment. Amyl nitrite 1 pearl every 2 minutes should be given until IV access is established. Then give sodium nitrite 300 mg IV over 3 to 5 minutes followed by sodium thiosulfate 12.5 g IV over 10 minutes. The above should be given where Cn toxicity is clinically suspected, because serum levels usually are not immediately available. These antidotes all can cause severe hypotension, so monitor BP closely. In combined CO and CN poisonings, nitrites (which cause a methemoglobinemia) should be withheld, but sodium thiosulfate can be given.

SPECIFIC ANTIDOTES

Table 10–1 presents a list of specific antidotes that are available for some of the more common poisonings not covered elsewhere in this chapter.

DISPOSITION

Factors that will affect your decision regarding disposition include:

- Clinical manifestations: Symptomatic patients should be admitted for observation. Unstable patients should be admitted to a monitored unit.
- Pharmacokinetics of the specific toxin: The onset, peak action, and duration of the agent all must be taken into account. Obviously, if the time elapsed since the ingestion is greater than the duration of the ingested toxin, it is safe to discharge the asymptomatic patient.
- Suicidal or homicidal ideation: Any patient who continues to be a threat to himself or oth-

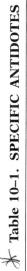

✳ Table 10–1. SPECIFIC ANTIDOTES

Toxin	Antidote	Comments
Cholinergic agents	Atropine 2 mg IV (0.05 mg/kg in children) q 10–30 minutes Pralidoxime 1 g IV for organophosphate poisonings	Give for **DUMBBELSS** syndrome; continue until respiratory secretions stop
Beta-blockers	Glucagon 3–10 mg IV over 2 minutes, then 2–4 mg/h	Give for bradycardia, heart block, or refractory hypotension
Nitrites	Methylene blue 1–2 mg/kg over 5 minutes	Give for coma, angina, or methemoglobin > 30%; exchange transfusion may be required
Heavy metals	Dimercaprol 3–5 mg/kg IM q 4 hours	Penicillamine or dimercaptosuccinic acid for mild cases
Benzodiazepines	Flumazenil 1–3 mg IV	Give 0.2 mg q 60 seconds to reverse life-threatening effects

DUMBBELSS: D = defecation; **U** = urination; **M** = miosis; **B** = bradycardia; **B** = bronchospasm; **E** = emesis; **L** = lacrimation; **S** = secretions; **S** = seizures; **IM** = intramuscularly; **IV** = intravenously.

ers should be evaluated by a psychiatrist or admitted with constant observation.

All patients with a potentially serious overdose should be observed for at least 6 hours before discharge or transfer to a nonmedical unit.

Some of the delayed-reacting substances that require more than 6 hours of observation can be remembered by the mnemonic **WAIT:**

W = warfarin
A = acetonitrile
I = industrial paint stripper (methylene chloride)
T = toxic cyanogenic plants and serious mushroom poisonings

11
CHAPTER

Obstetric and Gynecologic Problems

In this chapter we will present the two major problems seen in the ED that are specific to women: pelvic pain and vaginal bleeding. As an emergency physician, emphasis should be placed on recognizing conditions that can threaten a patient's life or fertility. In particular, you must rapidly assess the patient's hemodynamic stability and, if it is compromised, initiate resuscitative efforts while facilitating timely gynecologic consultation. Also you must determine whether or not the patient is pregnant. Therefore, all women of childbearing age should have a pregnancy test (preferably a serum beta human chorionic gonadotropin [hCG] test). Pelvic ultrasound, both transabdominal and transvaginal, is an extremely helpful diagnostic tool for delineating adnexal and uterine pathology and should be used in conjunction with gynecologic consultation whenever indicated.

PELVIC PAIN

In addition to considering all of the diagnostic possibilities discussed in the chapter on abdominal pain, emphasis should be placed on ruling out potentially life-threatening conditions, such as an ectopic pregnancy, a ruptured hemorrhagic ovarian cyst, or a ruptured tubo-ovarian abscess. Early recognition and treatment of an ectopic pregnancy can be life saving and can help prevent infertility and recurrences. Always assume that a woman of childbearing age is pregnant until proven otherwise. Studies show that 37% of pregnant women deny being pregnant when asked, and that 10% of women with normal menses who denied having any sexual activity and who stated that there was no chance that they were pregnant were found to be pregnant. Furthermore, 4% of women who were using birth control were found to be pregnant.

History

Include the following information in the patient's history:

- Prior pregnancy, abortion, miscarriage, and live births
- Details of associated abdominal pain (location, radiation, aggravating and relieving factors) or gastrointestinal symptoms such as nausea, vomiting, or diarrhea
- The temporal relation of the pain to menses and coitus
- A detailed menstrual history, including the regularity and specific details of the last two to three menstrual periods
- Associated urinary frequency or dysuria
- Associated vaginal itch, discharge, bleeding, or spotting
- Sexual practices and the use of contraception
- Prior history of sexually transmitted diseases
- Prior history of ectopic pregnancy
- History of dizziness or lightheadedness

Physical Examination

Vital Signs

Orthostatic as well as supine vital signs should always be measured. If the patient is unstable, rapidly establish venous access and give fluids. Notify Ob-Gyn as soon as possible. Send blood for type and cross and for beta hCG, and spin a hematocrit (see the following section on Laboratory Tests). If patient is in shock, give O-negative blood.

Pelvic Examination

All women of childbearing age with abdominal pain and all women with pelvic pain should have a formal pelvic exam. Inspection of the external genitalia for evidence of skin lesions should be performed before you insert a vaginal speculum. Lubricants facilitate the ease of the examination, but they have a bacteriostatic effect. Therefore, if you suspect infection use warm water as a lubricant. Note the presence of any lesions or sources of bleeding. Is the external cervical os open or closed? Is there any blood or discharge from the cervix? Are there any lesions on the cervix itself?

Next perform a bimanual examination. Evaluate for cervical motion tenderness; uterine size, tenderness, and consistency; and the presence of adnexal masses or tenderness.

It is best to always obtain cervical cultures for gonococci and chlamydia while performing the exam with a speculum. If an abnormal discharge or abnormal findings on bimanual exam are noted, you should also obtain a Venereal Disease Research Laboratory (VDRL) test. Wet smears of any abnormal cervical discharge should be viewed under a microscope for the presence of trichomonads (see Fig. 13–3), clue cells (see Fig. 13–5) (bacteria-coated epithelial cells suggestive of *G.*

vaginalis), or the spores and pseudohyphea of *C. albicans* ("meatballs and spaghetti" appearance [see Fig. 13–4]). The latter are demonstrated after dissolving the epithelial cells in KOH 10% solution. The presence of a "fishy" odor on adding KOH to the smear suggests the presence of bacterial vaginosis.

Laboratory Tests

In the presence of pelvic pain, the following laboratory tests are recommended: a serum beta hCG, CBC, electrolytes, glucose, BUN, creatinine, urinalysis, and cervical cultures. In cases of hemodynamic compromise, obtain a rapid assessment of the hematocrit by spinning a "crit." Spin a blood-filled micropipette for 60 seconds in a miniature centrifuge, and obtain the hematocrit by dividing the height of RBCs by the total height of the column. An erythrocyte sedimentation rate may be helpful when pelvic inflammatory disease (PID) is considered.

Specific Conditions Causing Pelvic Pain

Ectopic Pregnancy

Ectopic pregnancy occurs in 1% to 2% of all pregnancies. Risk factors include:

- A history of PID
- Prior history of an ectopic pregnancy
- Previous pelvic surgery
- History of tubal sterilization
- Use of an intrauterine contraceptive device
- History of induced abortions

Classically, the patient presents with a short period of amenorrhea followed by pain and abnormal bleeding. The pain usually is unilateral, but it may be diffuse and may or may not precede bleeding. Unilateral lower quadrant tenderness is common, although the patient may have a normal exam. Unilateral adnexal tenderness or a mass may be found. The uterus may be of normal size and, if enlarged, is usually smaller than expected by date of pregnancy.

In about 10% of cases, the ectopic pregnancy ruptures and significant intraperitoneal bleeding occurs; the patient may present with syncope, shock, or signs of peritoneal irritation. Shoulder pain, especially in the supine position, may be due to diaphragmatic irritation from intraperitoneal bleeding. A positive pregnancy test confirms the presence of a pregnancy, either intrauterine or ectopic. If the patient is unstable, immediate surgery is required, often before the results of the pregnancy test are available.

In all cases of suspected ectopic pregnancy, IV access with two large-bore angiocatheters should be established. The Ob-Gyn consultant should be involved as early as possible to expedite diagnosis and management. In the stable patient, pelvic ultrasound (abdominal or intravaginal) should be performed to look for an intrauterine gestational sac (which usually rules out an ectopic pregnancy) as well as adnexal masses or sacs. A gestational sac usually is evident by 4 to 5 weeks, a fetal pole by 5 to 6 weeks, and fetal heart motion by 6 to 7 weeks. The results of quantitative beta hCG, when available, are extremely helpful. An intrauterine pregnancy should be present on intravaginal ultrasound when the beta hCG level is > 1500 to 2000 mIU/L. Absence of a gestational sac on intravaginal ultrasound in a patient with a beta hCG above this discriminatory zone is highly suggestive of an ectopic pregnancy. Knowledge of your laboratory's threshold for detecting beta hCG is crucial for appropriate interpretation. Most labs will be able

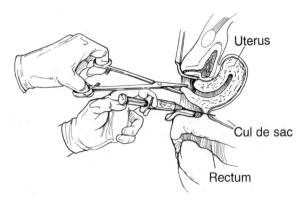

Figure 11–1. Culdocentesis. The posterior cervical lip is grasped with a tenaculum while blood is aspirated from the cul de sac.

to detect a level > 25 mIU/L in the serum and > 50 mIU/L in the urine. Rapid administration of fluids or a dilute urine can reduce the test's sensitivity.

If the patient is unstable, perform a culdocentesis to determine the presence of nonclotting blood. (A negative culdocentesis, while ruling out hemoperitoneum, does not exclude the possibility of an extrauterine pregnancy.) To perform a culdocentesis, insert a vaginal speculum and grab the posterior cervical lip with a tenaculum. Insert a # 18 spinal needle attached to a 10-mL syringe through the posterior fornix into the cul de sac (Fig. 11–1). To avoid uterine penetration, you should continuously pull back on the plunger till you get a free flow of fluid or blood, indicating entry into the peritoneal cavity. Aspiration of > 5 to 10 mL of nonclotting blood is evidence of intraperitoneal hemorrhage.

Ovarian Torsion

Ovarian torsion usually occurs in the presence of ovarian or fallopian pathology. Patients present with sudden onset of unilateral pain, which may be sharp or dull, constant or intermittent. Patients usually are afebrile. Physical examination reveals unilateral lower quadrant tenderness with or without signs of peritonitis. Most patients have unilateral adnexal tenderness and a mass, as well as some cervical motion tenderness.

The differential diagnosis includes unilateral PID, acute appendicitis, and ectopic pregnancy. If you suspect ovarian torsion, early gynecologic consultation and pelvic ultrasound should be performed.

Ovarian Cysts

Ovarian cysts are very common and often are asymptomatic. Symptomatic cysts usually are secondary to rupture, torsion, infection, or bleeding. Ovarian cysts may be *functional* (follicular or corpus luteum), *benign* (dermoid, teratoma), or *malignant*. Patients with a ruptured ovarian cyst usually present with a sudden onset of unilateral, sharp pelvic pain, often after exertion or coitus. On exam, patients are afebrile and may show signs of hemodynamic instability. Unilateral adnexal tenderness or a mass together with signs of peritoneal irritation may be present. Mittelschmerz occurs at midcycle in up to 25% of women due to rupture of a follicular cyst at the time of ovulation, and presents with unilateral pelvic pain lasting hours to several days.

Most small ovarian masses, especially if they enlarge before ovulation or menstruation, are benign. However, women with an adnexal mass should be reassessed by a gynecologist after their menses. All patients with signs of peritoneal irritation or hemodynamic instability must be seen urgently by a gynecologist.

Pelvic Inflammatory Disease

In PID, the pain often is bilateral and accompanied by bilateral adnexal tenderness, cervical discharge, and prominent cervical motion tenderness. Patients who are discharged should be treated with ceftriaxone 250 mg IM followed by doxycycline 100 mg PO bid and metronidazole 500 mg PO bid for 10 to 14 days. PID is discussed in more detail in Chapter 13 on sexually transmitted diseases (STDs).

Endometriosis

Endometriosis is the result of the abnormal location of endometrial tissue outside of the uterus (usually in the pelvis). Classically, the patient is in her late twenties or early thirties and presents with a combination of the following symptoms: *dysmenorrhea* (pain around menses), *dyspareunia* (pain during sexual intercourse), *menstrual abnormalities,* and *infertility.* Pain usually is bilateral, dull, and becomes progressively worse toward the end of the menstrual cycle. Bladder or bowel involvement can cause symptoms related to function of these organs. Rarely, sensitive nodules can be palpated on pelvic or rectal exam. The stable patient with presumed endometriosis should be referred to a gynecologist for consideration of hormonal therapy (danazol). Pain can be managed with NSAIDs.

VAGINAL BLEEDING

The Normal Menses

The average age of menarche is 12 years; the average age of onset of menopause is 48 years. The length of the menstrual cycle varies from 18 to 40 days. Bleeding is heaviest during the first 2 days and lasts 3 to 7 days. The average blood loss is 25 to 60 mL. The degree of blood loss can be estimated from the number of pads or tampons needed. An average tampon absorbs as much as 20 to 30 mL of blood.

Initial Assessment of Vaginal Bleeding

When a women presents with vaginal bleeding, two questions must be answered as soon as possible:

1. Is the vaginal bleeding causing hemodynamic compromise?
2. Is the patient pregnant?

Rapid assessment of the patient's ABCs, as well as orthostatic changes in the BP and pulse, should be measured as soon as possible. If the patient has evidence of hemodynamic compromise, immediately establish IV access with two large-bore IV catheters and initiate fluid resuscitation. Blood should be sent for a blood type and cross, CBC, platelets, PT, PTT, and a serum beta hCG. Have the blood bank type and cross-match 4 U of PRBCs. A gynecologist should be involved as soon as possible. Hemorrhaging can be controlled by packing the vagina with sterile towels until the operating room is available.

Vaginal Bleeding in the Nonpregnant Woman

Dysfunctional bleeding, usually secondary to a nonovulatory cycle, is the most common cause of vaginal bleeding in women of childbearing age. This is commonly seen around menarche or menopause, but may occur at any point in the cycle; it rarely leads to hemodynamic compromise. Most hemodynamically stable patients without significant anemia can be discharged safely from the hospital with early follow-up by a gynecologist. If bleeding is profuse but the patient is hemodynamically stable and has a hematocrit within normal limits, medroxyprogesterone (Provera, The Upjohn Company, Kalamazoo, MI) 10 mg PO qid for 10 days or conjugated estrogens tablets (Premarin, Wyeth-Ayerst Laboratories, Philadelphia, PA) 2.5 mg PO qid for 21 days followed by medroxyprogesterone for the last 5 days can be given in consultation with a gynecologist.

Other causes of vaginal bleeding in the nonpregnant woman include *neoplasms* and *trauma*. A thorough pelvic exam will pick up many of these illnesses, which will need gynecologic follow-up. A *generalized coagulopathy* should be suspected when a patient has a personal or family history of a bleeding tendency (blood in urine or stool, bleeding from gums, or easy bruising) and is evaluated with a PT, PTT, and a platelet count. Postmenopausal bleeding always should be presumed to be caused by neoplasms until proven otherwise. In children, suspect *foreign bodies* or *sexual abuse*.

Vaginal Bleeding in Early Pregnancy

First-trimester bleeding may be due to any of the causes of vaginal bleeding in the nonpregnant woman, as well as to a spontaneous abortion, an ectopic pregnancy, or gestational trophoblastic disease.

Patients having *spontaneous abortions* present with painless vaginal bleeding sometimes followed by crampy abdominal pain; bleeding preceded by pain is more characteristic of ectopic pregnancy. Perform an abdominal examination to

Table 11-1. DIFFERENTIATING PLACENTAL ABRUPTION FROM PLACENTA PREVIA

Parameter	Placental Abruption	Placenta Previa
Vaginal bleeding	Dark red, purple	Bright red
Pain	Severe	Absent or minimal
Uterine tenderness	Significant	Absent
Degree of shock	Out of proportion to external bleeding	Proportional to degree of external bleeding
Risk factors	Advanced maternal age and parity	Multiparity
	Maternal hypertension	Prior cesarean section
	Smoking history	

assess for tenderness or signs of peritoneal irritation. On the pelvic exam, note whether the external cervical os is open or closed and whether any clots or fetal tissue are evident. Microscopic evaluation of any passed tissue (in saline suspension) may show feathery-appearing chorionic villi.

Anti-D immune globulin (RhoGAM, Ortho Diagnostic Systems, a Johnson & Johnson Co., Raritan, NJ) 300 μg IM should be considered if the patient is Rh-negative; this will protect against a fetal–maternal hemorrhage of up to 30 mL. Ob-Gyn consultation should be obtained in all cases of abortion whether threatened, incomplete, or complete. Usually the patient will require a formal dilation and curettage.

Vaginal Bleeding in Later Pregnancy

Vaginal bleeding during the third trimester is usually caused by either *placental abruption* or *placenta previa*. As always, assess the ABCs and determine the hemodynamic stability of the patient. Two large-bore IV catheters should be established, and blood should be sent for type and cross, CBC, platelets, PT, PTT, fibrinogen, and fibrin split products (the latter to assess for disseminated intravascular coagulation [DIC] associated with placental abruption).

In the presence of placenta previa, a pelvic examination can cause catastrophic bleeding. Therefore, *avoid manual pelvic exams in patients with vaginal bleeding during late pregnancy*. Assessment for fetal heart tones should be made with a portable Doppler, and once the patient is stable she should be transferred to the delivery suite for further evaluation and management. Emergent pelvic ultrasound is extremely helpful in excluding a placenta previa. Table 11–1 distinguishes placental abruption from placenta previa.

12

CHAPTER

Common Pediatric Problems

This chapter covers selected topics in emergency pediatrics and includes some useful tricks and methods that will help you in dealing with the sick child. Although it is a cliché, this phrase bears repeating: "Children are not just little adults." Some techniques, such as intubation, are somewhat different in children. Vital signs differ by age. Some diseases, such as epiglottitis, present almost exclusively in children, and of course drug doses and equipment sizes must be scaled appropriately. This chapter also includes sections on two specific pediatric problem areas: the airway and fever. The last section of the chapter covers the topic of sedation.

GENERAL CONSIDERATIONS

In most cases, you'll have time to calculate drug dosages based on the child's weight. For situations in which this is not possible, as in a code, there are several approximation methods that are useful. The Broselow tape is a measuring device that every ED should have; to use it, merely measure the child's length with it, and then read off the proper

Table 12–1. NORMAL VITAL SIGNS BY AGE

Age	Respirations*	Pulse†	Systolic BP (mm Hg)
Newborn	40	140–160	60
3–6 months	30–40	120–140	80
1 year	20–30	110–130	90–100
5 years	20	100–110	100
8 years	12–20	90–100	105

*In breaths per minute.
†In beats per minute.
BP = blood pressure.

drug doses and equipment sizes. When this tape is not available you will have to estimate the weight: a 1-year-old infant weighs approximately 10 kg and a 5-year-old child approximately 20 kg. For children between the ages of 1 and 8, a useful formula is as follows:

$$\text{Weight (kg)} = (\text{age} \times 2) + 8.$$

You should practice estimating weights with all the children you see.

Normal vital signs do vary by age. Table 12–1 is a rough guide. The following is a useful formula for estimating minimum systolic BP:

$$70 + (\text{age} \times 2)$$

Children tend to compensate well for illnesses until the moment of collapse. An adult who loses 25% of his blood volume will be hypotensive, but a child with similar losses would show tachycardia but probably a preserved BP until the time he arrests. The lesson is that you must pay attention to the child's clinical appearance: in children, even more than in adults, what the patient "looks like" is the best indicator of clinical status. This judgment only comes with experience; try to develop it while you are in the ED. Use the level of the child's play-fulness in the ED as an indicator. In children, it often is helpful to assess capillary refill by pressing on the nail bed and measuring how long it takes for the color to return (it normally takes approximately 2 seconds). A capillary refill greater than 3 to 4 seconds suggests poor peripheral perfusion.

Pediatric codes tend to frighten and even "paralyze" novice clinicians. People may tend to focus on one task, such as attempting IV access, to the exclusion of taking care of the patient. Therefore, in addition to the ABCs, we offer you the "Seven Points of Light," or seven things that should be done for every pediatric code (note that none of them is IV access):

1. Oxygen.
2. History: Assign someone to gather this information from the persons who brought the child in.
3. Physical exam: Look for signs of trauma or petechial rash (possible sepsis).
4. Temperature—measured rectally. Look for hypothermia and fever.
5. Heel-stick blood for spun hematocrit.
6. Heel-stick blood for glucose chemstrip.
7. Cardiac monitor leads.

You should also, of course, intubate the patient and obtain IV or intraosseous access.

Fluid management for children in the emergency setting is simpler than longer-term calculations. In general, any dehydrated child should receive a bolus of normal saline of 20 mL/kg IV. This should be repeated until vital signs stabilize. Note, though, that if the child's volume loss is due to bleeding, you should give PRBCs at 10 mL/kg after the second fluid bolus. The degree of dehydration (*not* blood volume loss) can be estimated based on clinical signs. A child with mild (5%) dehydration has dry mucous membranes but otherwise appears normal. At a moderate (10%) level, the child is also tachycardic, with sunken eyeballs and fontanelle, and may be hypotensive. Severe (15%) dehydration is accompanied by additional symptoms of poor skin turgor, an altered sensorium, metabolic acidosis, poor capillary refill, and frank hypotension.

Once the patient is stable, you will need to calculate maintenance fluid requirements. An easy formula is as follows:

4 mL/kg per hour for the first 10 kg of weight
2 mL/kg per hour for the next 10 kg
1 mL/kg per hour for every kilogram thereafter

For example, a 23-kg child would require maintenance fluid as follows:

$$(4 \times 10) + (2 \times 10) + (1 \times 3) = 63 \text{ mL/h.}$$

The usual fluid for children under 10 kg is D_5W in 0.25 NS (Isolyte P with 5% Dextrose, American McGaw, Santa Ana, CA). For children over 10 kg, use $D_5W/0.5$ NS. In the setting of dehydration, the deficit also needs to be replaced; for hypotonic (hyponatremic) and isotonic dehydration, NS usually is given over a 24-hour period. For hypertonic (hypernatremic) dehydration, replacement fluid (usually D_5W) must be given over 48 hours to avoid cerebral edema. Note that the child should be receiving maintenance fluid as well during this period.

Some useful information on pediatric immunizations and oral drug dosing can be found in Tables 12–2 and 12–3.

THE PEDIATRIC AIRWAY

Adults tend to die cardiac deaths; children tend to die respiratory deaths. Supporting a child's res-

Table 12–2. PEDIATRIC IMMUNIZATION SCHEDULES

Age	Immunizations
Birth	HBV
2 months	DTP, HbCV, OPV, HBV
4 months	DTP, HbCV, OPV
6 months	DTP, HbCV, HBV
15 months	MMR, HbCV
15–18 months	DTP, OPV
4–6 years	DTP, OPV
4–12 years	MMR
14–16 years	Td

DTP = diphtheria, tetanus, and pertussis vaccine; HbCV = *H. influenzae* conjugate vaccine; HBV = hepatitis B vaccine; MMR = measles, mumps, and rubella vaccine; OPV = oral polio vaccine; Td = tetanus and diphtheria adult formulation vaccine.

piratory status often is the deciding factor in saving his or her life. Intubation of a child, while essentially the same procedure as in an adult, has some quirks. Tube size depends on the age of the child; use the following formula to estimate it:

$$\text{Tube size (mm)} = \frac{\text{child's age} + 16}{4}$$

Children's tubes (up to size 6, about age 5) are uncuffed because, unlike in an adult, the tightest area of the airway is subglottic. It also tends to be easier to use a straight (Miller) laryngoscope blade because a child's epiglottis is longer and floppier, and more anterior, than an adult's. Also because of a child's smaller size, it's easier to intubate the right mainstem bronchus, so be wary of this, and try to avoid passing the tube too deep. The distance from the teeth to the carina can be estimated by the following formula:

Table 12–3. COMMON PEDIATRIC ORAL DRUG DOSES

Generic Name (Brand Name)	Formulation	Dose
Acetaminophen (Tylenol)	80 mg/0.8 mL 160 mg/5 mL 80-mg chewtab	15 mg/kg q 4 hours
Ibuprofen (Pediaprofen)	100 mg/5 mL	10 mg/kg q 6 hours
Albuterol (Proventil)	2 mg/5 mL	2–5 years: 0.1 mg/kg tid 6–11 years: 2 mg tid 12+ years: 2 mg tid–qid
Prednisone (Pediapred)	5 or 25 mg/5 mL	2 mg/kg/day
Amoxicillin (Amoxil)	125 mg/5 mL 250 mg/5 mL	10 mg/kg tid

Penicillin V potassium (Pen·Vee K)	125 mg/5 mL 250 mg/5 mL	10 mg/kg qid
Cephalexin (Keflex)	125 mg/5 mL 250 mg/5 mL	10 mg/kg qid
Trimethoprim-sulfamethoxazole (Bactrim, Septra)	TMP 40 mg and SMX 200 mg/5 mL	Based on TMP as TMP 4 mg/kg bid By weight: 8 kg: 2.5 mL qid 16 kg: 5 mL qid 24 kg: 7.5 mL qid >45 kg: 10 mL qid
Erythromycin-sulfamethoxazole (Pediazole)	200 mg EM and 600 mg SMX/5 mL	

EM = erythromycin; SMX = sulfamethoxazole; TMP = trimethoprim.

$$\text{Distance (cm)} = \frac{\text{child's age}}{2} + 12.$$

Try not to hyperextend the neck, as this will bring the larynx even more anterior and complicate the intubation. At the end of the endotracheal tube are two black stripes. The first stripe should be passed beyond the vocal cords; leave the second stripe above the cords, which will ensure that the tube is always in place. The hardest part of intubation is ensuring that the tube stays in place—holding it and securing it with tape is essential! If you're having difficulty with intubation, consider doing a digital intubation after visualizing or palpating the epiglottis.

Epiglottitis

Because of the small size of a child's airway, a disease such as epiglottitis can be rapidly life-threatening. Typically, a child with this infectious disorder will present with a high fever, "toxic" (i.e., very sick) appearance, drooling, and sitting up on both arms (the "tripod" position). The voice is often muffled. When you suspect this diagnosis, do not agitate the child or put anything in his or her mouth, as this can cause acute airway obstruction by provoking laryngospasm. Immediately notify the operating room, anesthesiologist, and ENT or pediatric surgeon. Usually, the next step is to take the patient immediately to the operating room and do a mask induction with inhalational anesthetics, followed by intubation. Even starting an IV is best deferred until the airway is secured, because this can easily agitate the child. If the child blocks off his airway, all attempts at intubation must be done in the ED. If you have a low suspicion for epiglottitis and the child is stable, you can take a lateral neck x-ray of the soft tissues; epiglottitis is evidenced by a "thumbprint" (i.e., swollen) epiglottis. With the recent introduction of an effective vaccine for *H. influenzae* B, cases of epiglottitis are seen much less frequently, yet should never be missed.

Croup

Croup is another common pediatric airway problem. It is an infectious disease, a laryngotracheobronchitis usually caused by parainfluenza virus. In general, croup is not life-threatening and can be treated easily with humidified oxygen and occasionally corticosteroids (dexamethasone 0.3 mg/kg IM). The main difficulty is in distinguishing it from epiglottitis, but this usually can be accomplished on clinical grounds, as shown in Table 12–4. Children who are ill-appearing without having evidence of epiglottitis may have tracheitis, which can be quite serious and would require admission especially for pulmonary toilet. Severe respiratory distress can be treated with nebulized racemic epinephrine 0.25 to 0.5 mL. All patients receiving racemic epinephrine should be admitted or observed for at least 4 to 6 hours before discharge because rebound is common.

Asthma

Asthma is an extremely common pediatric problem consisting of reversible bronchospasm usually caused by allergies or concurrent infection. The mainstay of management is nebulized beta-adrenergic agonists such as albuterol or metaproterenol. The usual dose of albuterol is 2.5 mg in 2 mL of saline nebulized every 20 minutes until the attack is broken. Many studies show that this drug

Table 12–4. CROUP VERSUS EPIGLOTTITIS

	Croup	Epiglottitis
Age	6 months to 5 years; peak 2 years	3 to 6 years
Sex	M > F, 2:1	M = F
Season	Fall and winter	Variable
Etiology	Viral, usually parainfluenza	Bacterial, usually *H. influenzae* B
Prodrome	Upper respiratory infection	Usually none
Onset	Gradual	Rapid
Fever	Low-grade	High
Toxic?	No	Yes
Sore throat?	Variable	Yes
Voice	Hoarse	Muffled
Drooling?	No	Yes
Cough	Barking, "croupy"	No
Position	Variable	Prefers sitting or "tripod" position
WBC count*	Normal	High
Blood culture*	Negative	Positive
Lateral neck x-ray	"Steeple sign"	"Thumbprint" epiglottis

*Caution: In suspected epiglottitis, do not draw blood or do anything to agitate the patient until the ENT and anesthesia teams are ready to manage the patient's airway (usually in the operating room).
ENT = ear, nose, and throat; F = female; M = male; WBC = white blood cell.

also may be given continuously for 1 hour with relatively few side effects. To document improvement, we like to follow peak flow readings in children old enough to cooperate; this is especially useful in patients with known baseline peak flow values. Pulse oximetry also is helpful; it also can warn of hypoxia, which indicates the need for admission. Our standard method of treatment is to give the child three nebulizer treatments and then reassess. If there still is slight wheezing or slightly reduced peak flow but the child seems well, we discharge the child on beta-agonists and steroids, such as prednisone 2 mg/kg per day. If the child is completely back to normal, we may forgo the steroids. Indications for getting a chest x-ray include:

- A first episode of wheezing
- Fever
- Asymmetric lung exam
- Chest pain
- Hypoxia
- An intractable attack (requiring more than three nebulizer treatments)
- Hospital admission

Indications for hospital admission include:

- Hypoxia
- Intractable attack
- Concurrent pneumonia

In the most severe attacks, when patients are not responding to standard therapy, you may try systemic epinephrine (0.01 mg/kg up to 0.3 mg SC), theophylline (5 to 6 mg/kg bolus IV over 20 minutes followed by a continuous drip of 0.5 to 0.8 mg/kg per hour), magnesium sulfate, or ketamine. Patients in respiratory failure must be intubated.

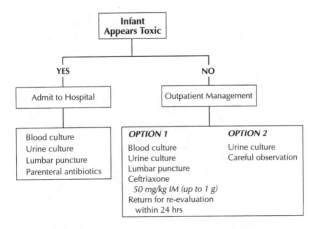

Figure 12–1. Management of a previously healthy low-risk infant aged 28 to 90 days old, with a fever without a source.

FEVER AND INFECTIOUS DISEASES

Although the most common cause of fever is a benign viral infection, a child younger than 2 years with fever can have such serious illnesses as meningitis or bacteremia without any obvious findings. Workup of fever in a child therefore depends on the child's age. At this point we will discuss the management of a child who has fever *without* a known source; if a focus of infection is found, treat the child as appropriate for that infection. The approaches discussed below have been suggested by a panel of pediatricians and emergency physicians who met to develop the American College of Emergency Physicians' guidelines and are summarized in Figures 12–1 and 12–2.

In the *newborn,* and up to 4 weeks of age, any fever warrants a full sepsis workup—in other words,

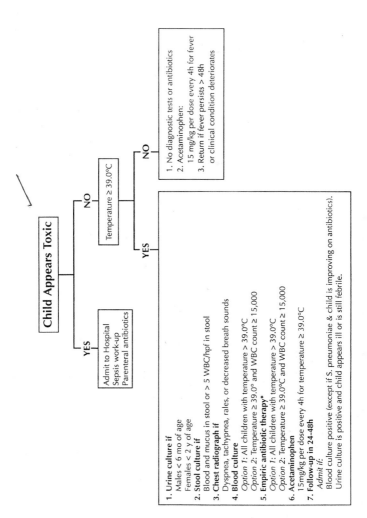

Child Appears Toxic

YES

Admit to Hospital
Sepsis work-up
Parenteral antibiotics

NO

Temperature ≥ 39.0°C

NO

1. No diagnostic tests or antibiotics
2. Acetaminophen:
   15 mg/kg per dose every 4h for fever
3. Return if fever persists > 48h
   or clinical condition deteriorates

YES

1. **Urine culture if**
   Males < 6 mo of age
   Females < 2 y of age
2. **Stool culture if**
   Blood and mucus in stool or > 5 WBC/hpf in stool
3. **Chest radiograph if**
   Dyspnea, tachypnea, rales, or decreased breath sounds
4. **Blood culture**
   Option 1: All children with temperature > 39.0°C
   Option 2: Temperature ≥ 39.0° and WBC count ≥ 15,000
5. **Empiric antibiotic therapy***
   Option 1: All children with temperature > 39.0°C
   Option 2: Temperature ≥ 39.0°C and WBC count ≥ 15,000
6. **Acetaminophen**
   15mg/kg per dose every 4h for temperature ≥ 39.0°C
7. **Follow-up in 24–48h**
   Admit if:
   Blood culture positive (except if S. pneumoniae & child is improving on antibiotics).
   Urine culture is positive and child appears ill or is still febrile.

Figure 12–2. Management of a previously healthy child, aged 3 to 24 months old, with a fever without a source.

FUO

blood culture, catheterized or suprapubic urine culture, lumbar puncture, and chest x-ray. The child should then be started on IV antibiotics, usually ampicillin 50 mg/kg IV every 8 hours and gentamicin 1.5 mg/kg IV every 8 hours, or cefotaxime 200 mg/kg per day IV in three divided doses, and hospitalized until culture results come back.

Children between *28 and 90 days* of age should be classified as *low risk* or *high risk*. A child is considered low risk if he or she meets *all* of the following criteria:

- Previously healthy
- Appears nontoxic
- No focal bacterial infection except otitis media
- Good social situation with reliable follow-up
- WBC count between 5000 and 15,000 with fewer than 1500 band forms
- Less than 5 WBC/high power field on urinalysis (catheterized or suprapubic sample)
- Less than 5 WBC/high power field in stool, if diarrhea present

This workup requires blood drawing for the CBC, so it is usually a good idea to draw blood for a culture at the same time, in case you decide to order one. This saves the child another needle stick. High-risk children are pan-cultured as above and admitted to the hospital. If the child is low risk, there are two generally accepted options (see Fig. 12–1). Which one you use will depend on your local protocols or clinical experience.

Option 1: Send a urine culture to the lab and discharge the child with close follow-up (i.e., to be seen again in the ED or by the primary pediatrician within 24 hours [*call* the pediatrician to let him or her know]). Warn the caregiver to bring the child back if *any* worsening occurs, and prescribe acetaminophen 15 mg/kg given orally or rectally every 4 hours for fever.

Option 2: Send a blood culture *and* perform an LP for CSF cell count and culture; then give the child ceftriaxone 50 mg/kg IM. This provides 24 hours of IV-equivalent antibiotic coverage. This child also *must* be seen again in 24 hours to receive another dose of ceftriaxone. If the blood and CSF cultures are negative at 48 hours, antibiotics then can be discontinued.

For children with fever who are between *12 weeks and 2 years* of age, discharge and close follow-up generally is acceptable if, and only if, the child appears clinically well (see Fig. 12–2). Some clinicians send off blood cultures as a screen for bacteremia, planning on calling the patient back if the cultures are positive. The argument has been made that a WBC count of 15,000 or higher is predictive of bacteremia and should be used as an indication for admission for administration of IV antibiotics. Unfortunately, whereas a WBC count this high may predict bacteremia, it only predicts pneumococcal bacteremia; children who have this infection, but look well, will do well regardless of antibiotics. Children with the far more serious *H. influenzae* bacteremia, who do need IV antibiotics, usually have normal WBC counts. We therefore cannot routinely rely on this lab value for admission decisions. We do recommend that all children up to 2 years old have a urine sample cultured for possible UTI, since this can result in severe kidney damage if untreated.

A few words should be said about *meningitis.* In children, as in adults, the most common etiology of meningitis is viral. Bacterial meningitis, however, is rightfully feared because of its high morbidity and mortality. Whenever you suspect meningitis, expedite the performance of the LP and administer IV antibiotics (cefotaxime 50 mg/kg) as soon as possible. In fact, if waiting for an LP will significantly delay therapy, draw blood cultures, and give the antibiotics. The CSF Gram's stain still will be accurate, and the blood cultures may very well grow out the offending organism. Also, immune electrophoresis for bacterial antigens will be positive despite any antibiotic use. Corticosteroid therapy has been shown to reduce complications (especially auditory) in *H. influenzae* meningitis, and it often is used for all cases of suspected bacterial meningitis. The usual initial dose is dexamethasone 0.15 mg/kg IV simultaneously with or even slightly before the first dose of antibiotics. If possible, you should discuss the use of steroids with the admitting pediatrician.

Children older than 2 or 3 years who have a fever (rectal temperature ≥ 38° C) can be evaluated as you would any other patients. They usually can tell you what hurts, and they will develop the characteristic physical findings of specific infectious illnesses. The single most important indicator of serious illness is how the child looks and interacts with his surroundings. A very common focal infection of young children is *otitis media*, and thus you always should examine the ears of any child you see. This disease is usually caused by pneumococcus or *H. influenzae* and treated with amoxicillin; if it has persisted despite this therapy, treatment with antibiotics such as trimethoprim/sulfamethoxazole or cephalosporins is warranted. Treatment for otitis media usually is continued for 10 days. The dosages of oral antibiotics are summarized in Table 12–3.

Sore throat is another common infectious complaint. Be aware that only streptococcal infection requires treatment with antibiotics (usually penicillin for 10 days), and then only to prevent rheumatic fever. In many cases, though, this diagnosis will require culture, which takes 1 to 2 days. Some physicians wait for culture results, and others treat presumptively. In general, your choice will depend on how certain you are that a follow-up appointment will be kept. Local customs or parental wishes often prevail.

Febrile seizures can be extremely frightening, but usually do not indicate meningitis or other serious disease. The mainstay of therapy is cooling, usually with antipyretics (e.g., acetaminophen and ibuprofen) or tepid baths. An LP to exclude meningitis often needs to be done, but can occasionally be spared. See Figure 12–3 for a summary of febrile seizure management.

A common question that parents have is, "Do I need to keep him home from school?" The general answer is that an infectious child should be kept isolated from others until the period of infectivity has passed. Table 12–5 summarizes isolation recommendations for some common and uncommon diseases to help you in giving parents advice.

PEDIATRIC SEDATION

The ideal sedative would be painless to administer, have a rapid onset of action, have no side effects or risks, and wear off as soon as it was no longer needed. Of course, no real drug meets all of these criteria. Due to the inconvenience and risks of sedation, many painful and frightening procedures are performed on children using "brutane" (i.e., physical force) to accomplish. Often, if you take the time to create a comfortable setting and reassure and distract the child, less force will be needed. In addition, we believe that if properly administered and monitored, and if used in the appropriate settings (i.e., in longer and more complex procedures), sedative drugs can be used safely to minimize a child's distress in most cases. Once a child has been sedated, he or she *must* be monitored until awake. Do not discharge any child until

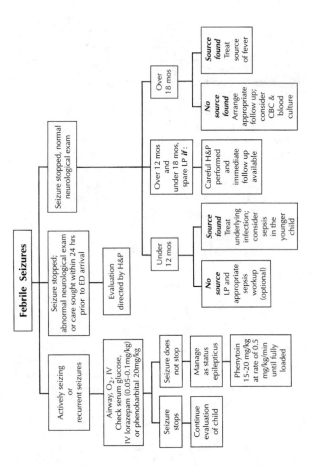

Figure 12–3. Approach to febrile seizures.

Table 12–5. PERIOD OF INFECTIVITY OF SELECTED DISEASES

Disease	Infectivity	Isolation
Chickenpox	From 1–2 days before rash appears to when all lesions are crusted (5–6 days)	From those who never had the disease, or who are immunocompromised, until all lesions crusted
Hepatitis A	1–3 weeks	Enteric precautions until asymptomatic and LFTs normal
Measles	1–2 days before rash appears until 4 days after rash appears	Respiratory isolation
Scarlet fever	Until 1–2 days of therapy complete	Until 24 hours after therapy started
Streptococcal pharyngitis	Until 1–2 days of therapy complete	Until 24 hours after therapy started

LFTs = liver function tests.

the sedative has worn off. A child sent home sedated is an invitation to disaster.

The most effective method of sedation is to use titratable IV agents such as midazolam 0.01 mg/kg IV and fentanyl 1 µg/kg IV. These doses are to be repeated every 5 to 10 minutes until sedation occurs. This requires the constant attendance at the bedside of a physician and nurse skilled in pediatric resuscitation, continuous cardiac and pulse oximetry monitoring, and the availability of pediatric resuscitation equipment. Therefore, this method can be used only rarely in a busy ED, although it is often the best method for orthopedic procedures or complex suturing.

For sedation for CT scans or other radiologic studies, we usually use secobarbital or pentobarbital 4 to 6 mg/kg IM. If the first dose does not produce adequate sedation, half of that amount can be repeated once, approximately 30 minutes after the first dose. These drugs induce 45 to 60 minutes of sedation and usually do not cause significant respiratory depression at these doses. Nevertheless, pediatric patients receiving these doses should be monitored continuously by pulse oximetry until the sedation wears off.

Ketamine 4 mg/kg IM or 1 mg/kg IV is a useful sedative because it does not abolish the gag reflex, and the airway thus remains relatively protected. It does produce increased secretions and should be preceded by atropine 0.01 mg/kg IV to reduce salivation. Ketamine produces dissociative amnesia: The child will appear awake but won't react to stimuli. It requires the same care and precautions as midazolam/fentanyl sedation. To avoid "reemergence nightmares," some physicians give diazepam 0.05 to 0.1 mg/kg IV or midazolam 0.01 mg/kg IV with the ketamine. Ketamine should be avoided in patients with upper airway disease or a psychiatric history.

Other drugs are used for pediatric sedation, but

Table 12–6. INITIAL ANTIBIOTIC THERAPY (FIRST DOSE) FOR POSSIBLE SEPSIS

Patient Characteristics	Drug	Dose (mg/kg)
Neonate (<1 month)	Ampicillin and cefotaxime	50 50
1 month–adolescent	Cefotaxime or ceftriaxone	50 50–100
Immunocompromised	Nafcillin and ceftazidime	50 30–50
Indwelling central line	Vancomycin and ceftazidime	10–15 30–50

Table 12–7. PEDIATRIC RESUSCITATION MODALITIES

Modality	Dose/Administration and Route
Epinephrine	0.01 mg/kg; IV, ET, IO
Atropine	0.02 mg/kg; IV, ET, IO (minimum 0.1 mg/dose)
Lidocaine	1 mg/kg; IV, ET, IO to maximum of 3 mg/kg
Defibrillation	2–4 J/kg; start at 2 J/kg; double with each shock to 4 J/kg maximum
Crystalloid	20 mL/kg; IV, IO (may repeat to a total of three boluses)

ET = endotracheal tube; IO = intraosseous; IV = intravenous.

we generally do not recommend them. A combination of Demerol (meperidine; Sanofi Winthrop Pharmaceuticals, New York, NY), Phenergan (promethazine; Wyeth-Ayerst Laboratories, Philadelphia, PA), and Thorazine (chlorpromazine; SmithKline Beecham Pharmaceuticals, Philadelphia, PA) (DPT) induces very deep and prolonged sedation and can cause dystonic reactions. Chloral hydrate is an unreliable agent; it can cause cardiac toxicity in some children even at normal doses. Regardless of the type of sedation chosen, be prepared for complications. All patients should be placed on a cardiac monitor and pulse oximetry and should be closely observed.

Tables 12–6 and 12–7 provide additional information that you will find useful when providing pediatric care.

13
CHAPTER

Common Infections

Despite the abundance of antibiotics today, infectious diseases are still common and often serious illnesses. In this chapter, we briefly review several of the more common infections encountered in the ED, covering the diagnostic workup, indications for referral or admission, and the initial choices involved in outpatient management.

Whenever indicated, appropriate microbiologic specimens should be obtained before you initiate therapy. The initial choice of antibiotics should be based on the most commonly infecting organisms and their local patterns of antimicrobial susceptibilities.

URINARY TRACT INFECTIONS

In women with classic symptoms of UTI, such as dysuria and urinary frequency, a positive leukocyte esterase and/or nitrates on a urine dipstick correlates highly with infection and justifies giving a course of antibiotics. In other patients, a urinalysis should be obtained. If your ED has a centrifuge and microscope, you can save a lot of time by spinning down the urine yourself (for 3 to 5 minutes) and observing the supernatant under high power field. The presence of >5 WBC/high power field

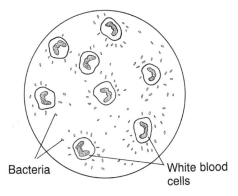

Bacteria

White blood cells

Figure 13–1. Typical microscopic findings in a urinary tract infection.

and/or bacteriuria in an unspun specimen are evidence of UTI (Fig. 13–1).

In men with symptoms of UTI, perform a rectal exam. (Avoid vigorous prostatic massage, which can cause bacteremia.) Tenderness or bogginess over the prostate gland suggests prostatitis.

A urine culture should be obtained in the following cases:

- All men and all children with UTI
- Patients with recurrent or persistent infections
- Patients with urosepsis or severe toxicity
- When the patient will be referred to a specialist

Patients should be referred to a urologist for further workup if they:

- Are young children
- Are men
- Have pyelonephritis
- Are women with frequent infections

In the past, much emphasis was put on differentiating upper UTIs (pyelonephritis) from lower

UTIs. Today, this distinction is less important in the ED because more patients with pyelonephritis are being managed as outpatients. Indications for admitting a patient with UTI include:

- Vomiting and dehydration unresponsive to oral rehydration
- Severe toxicity or sepsis
- Severe underlying diseases or immunocompromise (e.g., diabetes, steroids, chemotherapy)
- Pregnant women with pyelonephritis (order a pregnancy test in all women of childbearing age)
- Anatomic abnormalities of the urinary tract
- Fever and costovertebral angle tenderness in patients older than 50 years of age

Outpatient Management

Because the most common infecting organism is *E. Coli* and in most areas roughly 30% of *E. Coli* are resistant to ampicillin, we prefer an initial regimen of trimethoprim-sulfamethoxazole double-strength bid for 7 to 10 days. Alternatives include amoxicillin 500 mg PO tid or a second-generation cephalosporin such as cephalexin 500 mg PO qid. Ciprofloxacin and nitrofurantoin are other options. Women with a history of recurrent UTIs may be treated with a 3-day course of antibiotics if good follow-up is assured.

COMMUNITY-ACQUIRED PNEUMONIAS

Assessment

The majority of community-acquired pneumonias in the immunocompetent population are due to pneumococci, mycoplasma, or viruses. Often, the diagnosis may be made based on clinical impression alone (e.g., fever, chills, productive cough, localized evidence of consolidation). The diagnosis of mycoplasma pneumonia may be suggested by the presence of cold agglutinins. Several drops of blood should be added to a purple-topped, anticoagulated tube and then placed in ice water. If clumps (agglutinated blood) appear along the sides of the test tube when the tube is slowly tilted on its side, and the clumps dissolve on rewarming, cold agglutinins are present. The absence of cold agglutinins does not exclude the possibility of mycoplasma pneumonia.

Indications for a chest x-ray include:

- A low pulse oximetry reading
- Tachypnea or retractions
- Unclear diagnosis
- HIV infection
- The presence of rales (to exclude consolidation or effusion)

With the growing availability of pulse oximetry in most EDs, all patients with a diagnosis of pneumonia should have oximetry.

Disposition

Indications for admission include:

- Severe toxicity or sepsis
- Recurrent vomiting and dehydration
- Hypoxia requiring supplemental O_2 to maintain an O_2 saturation > 90% *or* a Po_2 > 70
- Severe underlying disease or immunocompromise (e.g., diabetes, COPD, CHF, malignancy)
- Poor social support and lack of good medical follow-up
- Extremes of age (infants and elderly)

- Failure of a trial of outpatient management
- Multilobar pneumonia or a pleural effusion
- High risk of tuberculosis

Management

Erythromycin 500 mg PO qid for 10 to 14 days probably is the best choice, covering both pneumococci and mycoplasma organisms. Better tolerated forms of erythromycin include E.E.S. Chewable Tablets 400 mg tid (Abbott Laboratories, Abbott Park, IL) or E-Mycin 250 mg qid (The Upjohn Company, Kalamazoo, MI). The newer macrolides (e.g., azithromycin 500 mg PO on the first day followed by 250 mg PO bid for 4 more days; clarithromycin 250 to 500 mg PO bid for 5 days) usually are better tolerated but more expensive. In the elderly, mycoplasma is less common and penicillin V potassium 500 mg PO qid for 10 days can be given.

SORE THROATS

The goals in managing a patient with a sore throat are to identify and treat streptococcal infection in order to avoid severe immunologic sequelae (e.g., rheumatic fever, glomerulonephritis), and to rule out life-threatening complications of pharyngeal infection.

Despite popular belief to the contrary, it is impossible to differentiate streptococcal infections from other causes of pharyngitis based on clinical grounds alone. Also, remember that most sore throats are caused by viral infections. Several epidemiologic and clinical factors increase the likelihood of streptococcal infection:

- Age > 5 years and < 15 years
- Household contacts who have streptococcal infection
- High fever, anterior cervical adenopathy, and tonsilar exudate
- Lack of signs and symptoms of systemic involvement (e.g., diffuse adenopathy, cough, runny nose, muscular aches and pains)

Even with all the above symptoms present, confirmation of streptococcal infections usually rests on a positive throat culture or a positive rapid streptococcal antigen assay. (These, too, can be inaccurate but are the best tools we have, short of serologic confirmation).

Management

A full 10-day course of antistreptococcal therapy, even without culture verification, is indicated in patients who have a history of rheumatic fever or rheumatic heart disease, recent exposure to a documented case of streptococcal infection, or a classic rash of scarlet fever.

In some hospitals, it is possible to obtain a rapid streptococcal antigen assay. A positive finding warrants antibiotic therapy without the need for a throat culture; however, a negative assay does not reliably rule out streptococcal infection and should be followed with a throat culture. If you have a high index of suspicion for streptococcal infection in patients whom you expect will have poor follow-up and compliance, a full 10-day course of therapy is warranted even without a throat culture. In patients with a good follow-up likelihood, you can postpone therapy until the results of the throat culture are known (usually in 2 days). If the patient appears very uncomfortable, you may want to start therapy in the ED and have the patient discontinue medication if the culture results are negative.

Penicillin V potassium 250 to 500 mg PO qid for 10 days is the most specific therapy. In penicillin-allergic patients, erythromycin 250 to 500 mg PO qid for 10 days is a good alternative. As the role of *Chlamydia*—recently reported in the etiology of pharyngitis—becomes clarified, erythromycin may become the therapy of choice for all patients.

Complications

Infection of the pharynx can extend into any of the potential surrounding spaces (peritonsillar, retropharyngeal, and prevertebral). If there is deep extension of the infection, urgent ENT consultation as well as hospital admission are required. Incision and drainage of abscesses and administration of IV antibiotics usually are indicated. Always ask the patient about difficulty breathing or swallowing (not pain on swallowing). Note whether there is cyanosis or any other evidence of upper airway obstruction, such as stridor.

Lateral x-rays of the soft tissues of the neck and/or direct fiberoptic laryngoscopy to rule out supraglottic or subglottic involvement should be performed in the stable patient with either of the following:

- A significant sore throat yet a relatively unimpressive pharyngeal exam
- The presence of voice changes (a voice with a "hot-potato" quality) or other evidence of upper airway obstruction

Maintaining a high index of suspicion in all cases of sore throat will help early identification and treatment of potentially life-threatening complications and adult epiglottitis.

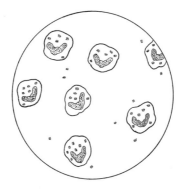

Figure 13–2. Gram-negative intracellular diplococci.

SEXUALLY TRANSMITTED DISEASES

Despite the increasing fear of contracting AIDS through sexual contact, promiscuity and STDs continue to be on the rise. On encountering a patient with an STD, take advantage of the opportunity to explain to the patient how sexual transmission of diseases may be avoided. Successful management will also require concurrent treatment of sexual partners to avoid reinfection.

Male patients usually present with purulent urethral discharge associated with dysuria. Female patients present with vaginal discharge, dysuria, and abdominal pain. However, infections may be asymptomatic in both sexes.

Historically, the most common STD has been *gonorrhea*. Recently, *chlamydia* has become increasingly prevalent. Often, concurrent infection with both organisms is present. Diagnosis is made by obtaining cultures and smears of abnormal genital discharge. A Gram's stain demonstrating Gram-negative intracellular diplococci is diagnostic of *Neisseria gonorrhoeae* (Fig. 13–2). Treatment

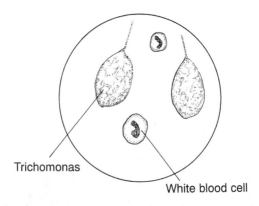

Trichomonas

White blood cell

Figure 13–3. A trichomonad seen in a wet smear at high power magnification.

with ceftriaxone 250 mg IM followed by doxycycline 100 mg PO bid for 7 days will cover both gonococci and chlamydia. One oral dose of azithromycin 1 g can be given alternatively for chlamydial coverage and guarantees compliance. A VDRL should be obtained in all such patients, since the above treatment is inadequate for syphilis. Chlamydia infections also can cause painless skin lesions (e.g., ulcers, papules, nodules, vesicles) or inguinal adenopathy.

Trichomonas vaginalis is characterized by copious, malodorous, foamy yellow-green vaginal discharge. Diagnosis is made microscopically by identification of the parasites on a wet smear (Fig. 13–3). Metronidazole 500 mg PO bid for 7 days or a single oral dose of metronidazole 2 g is used for treatment. Note, however, that metronidazole is contraindicated in pregnancy.

Candidiasis is characterized by a white, cheesy vaginal discharge, often with significant erythema and pruritis of the vulva and vagina. Spores or pseudohyphae can be seen on microscopy after application of 10% KOH to a smear of the discharge (Fig. 13–4).

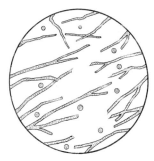

Figure 13–4. Candida albicans seen as spores and pseudohyphae in a KOH smear.

Bacterial vaginosis is characterized by a thin, gray, homogenous, malodorous discharge. Pruritis is uncommon; the discharge is increased by menses and intercourse. Typically, the addition of 10% KOH to a slide containing a discharge smear produces a fishy odor. Bacterial vaginosis is caused by a variety of bacteria, such as *G. vaginalis,* and is characterized by a vaginal pH>4.5. Diagnosis is supported by the presence of clue cells (epithelial cells with bacteria adherent to their borders [Fig. 13–5]). Treatment can be accomplished with 0.75% metronidazole vaginal gel applied twice daily for 5 days or with 2% clindamycin vaginal cream applied before bedtime for 7 days. The differential diagnosis of vaginal infections is presented in Table 13–1.

Pelvic Inflammatory Disease

It is important to identify and initiate treatment for PID as early as possible. This will decrease the possibility of extension of the infection as well as late complications such as ectopic pregnancy and infertility. PID often is polymicrobial, including gonococci, chlamydia, and anaerobic bacteria.

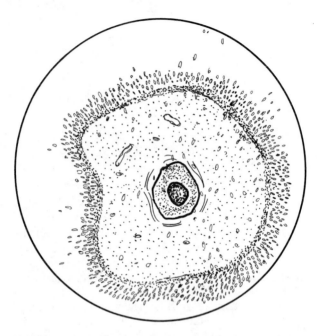

Figure 13–5. Clue cells characteristic of bacterial vaginosis. Note the epithelial cell coated with bacteria.

Criteria for the clinical diagnosis of PID include the presence of *all of the following:*

1. Abdominal tenderness with or without rebound tenderness
2. Cervical motion tenderness
3. Adnexal tenderness *plus* one of the following conditions:
   a. a positive Gram's stain from endocervical discharge
   b. fever $> 38°C$
   c. WBC $> 10,000/mL$

Indications for hospital admission include severe toxicity or sepsis and failure to respond to outpatient therapy.

Table 13–1. DIFFERENTIAL DIAGNOSIS OF VAGINAL INFECTIONS

	Normal	Bacterial Vaginosis	Trichomonas Vaginitis	Candida Vulvovaginitis
Vaginal pH	3.8–4.2	>4.5	>4.5	<4.5 (usually)
Discharge	White	Thin, homogenous, gray, adherent, increased	Yellow, frothy, adherent, increased	White, curdy, "cottage cheese"
KOH "whiff test"	Absent	Present (fishy)	May be present	Absent
Symptoms	None	Malodorous discharge, itching possibly present	Excessive discharge, foul odor, vulvar pruritis, dysuria	Itching/burning, discharge
Microscopy	Lactobacilli, epithelial cells	Clue cells, no WBCs	Trichomonads, WBCs >10/HPF	Budding yeast, hyphae, pseudohyphae

HPF = high power field; WBCs = white blood cells.

Outpatient management of PID should include:

1. Ceftriaxone 250 mg IM, *plus*
2. Doxycycline 100 mg PO bid, *or* tetracycline 500 mg PO qid, *or* ofloxacin 400 mg PO bid for 14 days, *plus*
3. Clindamycin 450 mg PO qid *or* metronidazole 500 mg PO bid for 14 days

If the patient is sent home, re-evaluation within 48 hours is necessary.

DIARRHEA

Diarrhea is defined as the rapid passage of poorly formed stools. Although in the United States this is a relatively benign disease, worldwide, it still is one of the leading causes of death. The causes of diarrhea are varied; in the ED, however, most cases involve patients with infectious, virally caused diarrhea.

The major complications of diarrhea are dehydration and hypovolemia. Therefore, emphasis should be placed on assessing the patient's hemodynamic status. Orthostatic changes in the pulse and BP, as well as the supine vital signs, need to be measured. Dry mucous membranes, poor skin turgor, thirst, and cool peripheral extremities are additional measures of dehydration.

History

Include the following information in the patient's history:

- Description of the character of the stool (e.g., presence of blood or mucous)
- Associated symptoms such as vomiting, fever, chills, and abdominal pain

- Epidemiologic factors: contact with patients with diarrhea, development of similar symptoms in people who shared the same meal
- Recent travel history
- Medication history (e.g., laxatives, antibiotics)

Always perform a rectal exam. Obtain a stool specimen and stain with methylene blue for evidence of fecal leukocytes. The presence of RBCs or WBCs suggests an invasive bacterial infection or inflammatory bowel diseases, and these tests should be followed by stool cultures for bacteria and a search for ova and parasites. X-rays usually are not helpful but may rule out toxic megacolon in patients with ulcerative colitis.

Management

Rehydration constitutes the cornerstone of ED management. Remember that oral rehydration often is all that is required. In fact, this is the most common form of treatment worldwide. If the patient is frankly hypotensive or is vomiting and unable to drink, establish IV access and give fluids as dictated by the clinical situation. For adults, D_5W lactated Ringer's solution or D_5W 0.45% NS with KCl 20 mEq/L and $NaHCO_3$ 50 mEq/L are additional options (considering the loss of bicarbonate and potassium in the stool). Note that KCl should be added to the fluids only after the patient voids. Antibiotics should be given rarely in the ED and should be based on specific stool culture results (in certain infections, such as salmonella, antibiotics actually can prolong the carrier state). Do not prescribe antispasmodic agents if invasive diarrhea is a possibility. Kaopectate or Pepto-Bismol can be given for severe cases. Arrange for a proper follow-up appointment and have the patient return to the ED if he or she is unable to drink fluids.

MENINGITIS

Despite the wide availability of highly efficacious antibiotics, the mortality and morbidity associated with bacterial meningitis remain high. Most cases of meningitis are caused by bacteria or viruses; fungi and parasites are less common etiologic agents. Epidemiologic factors such as age, season, and history of exposure to a patient with meningitis help predict the etiologic agents. *S. pneumoniae* and *N. meningitidis* are the most common causes of bacterial meningitis in the healthy adult. *H. influenzae* is more common in children younger than 5 years; *E. coli,* group B streptococci, and *L. monocytogenes* are seen most often in the newborn. Gram-negative rods and *L. monocytogenes* also are seen more frequently in alcoholic and immunosuppressed patients. Staphylococci should be considered in patients with a recent history of craniotomy. Early diagnosis and aggressive management are the keys to successful management. Therefore, all patients in whom the diagnosis of meningitis is entertained must have an immediate LP for CSF analysis.

History and Physical Examination

Classically, patients with meningitis present with fever, headache, vomiting, photophobia, seizures, and an alteration in the mental status. On examination, many patients will be found to have neck stiffness. Clinical signs and symptoms are not always reliable in distinguishing viral from bacterial meningitis, particularly at the extremes of age and in the immunocompromised patient. This distinction requires CSF analysis. Although rare, papilledema should always be sought. Its presence suggests an increase in ICP and warrants the performance of a head CT scan *before* LP; otherwise, herniation could result. CT of the head also should be obtained before LP in the presence of focal neurologic findings, severe alterations in the sensorium, seizures, evidence of recent head trauma, in patients with HIV infection, and in patients with an atypical or subacute presentation.

Lumbar Puncture

A LP should be performed at the level of the L3–5 interspaces. The L3–4 interspace is found directly above an imaginary line connecting the superior surfaces of the iliac crests. In patients who can sit, this often is the easiest position for an LP, although pressures obtained can be unreliable. The lateral decubitus or "fetal" position is more practical in the debilitated patient. If you are unsuccessful with the patient in one position, it often is helpful to try changing positions. Use of a small-gauge spinal needle (#20 to #22) will help minimize the incidence of headaches. At least three 1-mL tubes should be obtained. The first tube should be sent for a Gram's stain, culture and sensitivity, and bacterial antigens. The second tube should be sent for protein and glucose. (A serum glucose should be obtained simultaneously for comparison). The third tube should be sent for cell count and differential. The differential diagnosis of meningitis based on the CSF findings is presented in Table 13–2. A traumatic bloody tap can be distinguished from bloody CSF by the absence of xanthochromia in the supernatant after centrifugation. After a traumatic tap, the true WBC count can be estimated by subtracting 1 WBC for every 500 to 1000 RBCs. Similarly, the CSF protein can be corrected by subtracting 1 mg/dL for every 1000 RBCs. Contrary to wide belief, prior treatment with oral or parenteral antibiotics has a minimal effect on the

Table 13–2. CEREBROSPINAL FLUID FINDINGS

	Normal	Bacterial	Partially Treated Bacterial	Viral	Tuberculosis
Cells/mL	<5	200–5000	200–5000	<1000	<1000
Predominant cell type	Mononuclear	PMNs	PMNs	Mononuclear	Mononuclear
CSF/serum glucose ratio	0.6	Low	Low or normal	Normal	Low
Protein (mg/dL)	15–45	Very high	High	High	High
Gram's stain	Negative	Positive	Usually positive	Negative	Negative
Bacterial culture	Negative	Positive	May be positive	Negative	Negative

PMNs = polymorphonuclear leukocytes.

results of CSF analysis; however, cultures may be negative. Counter-immunoelectrophoresis for bacterial antigens (*H. influenzae, N. meningitidis,* and *S. pneumoniae*) is very useful and highly specific, but false-negatives are not uncommon. Bacterial antigens are particularly useful in cases of partially treated meningitis.

Management

As always, the ABCs need to be addressed initially. Active airway management, especially in the presence of seizures or altered mental status, often is required. Patients with hemodynamic compromise should be treated aggressively with IV fluids; avoid overhydration in stable patients. Patients with suspected bacterial meningitis should receive antibiotics as soon as possible. Antibiotics should never be withheld when LP is delayed (such as while awaiting the results of a head CT scan), but samples for blood cultures should be obtained before they are administered. Sterilization of spinal fluid is rare in the first 6 hours. In the absence of a specific etiologic agent, a third-generation cephalosporin, such as cefotaxime or ceftriaxone 2 g IV (50 mg/kg in children), is a good initial choice. In the neonate, ampicillin 50 mg/kg IV should be added for coverage of *L. monocytogenes.* The use of steroids, such as dexamethasone 0.15 mg/kg IV, can help prevent hearing loss if given early enough. Close contacts of patients with either meningococcal or *H. influenzae* meningitis should receive rifampin 600 mg PO (10 mg/kg in children) every 12 hours for 2 days.

All patients with suspected bacterial meningitis should be admitted and receive IV antibiotics pending culture results. Otherwise healthy patients with viral meningitis can be discharged if good follow up is ensured.

SEPTIC SHOCK

Septic shock, if not identified and treated early, is associated with a high rate of mortality. Septic shock should be suspected in any patient with a fever and hypotension, although sepsis may be present in the absence of a fever in the very young or old and in the immunocompromised patient.

The most common sources of septicemia are the genitourinary and gastrointestinal tracts. Therefore, Gram-negative rods are the predominant organisms; Gram-positive cocci, anaerobes, and fungi are other causes.

Management

Attention to the patient's ABCs is paramount. Septic shock usually is secondary to peripheral vasodilatation and may require large amounts of IV fluids. IV access should be established with at least two large-bore IV catheters, and patients should be placed on a cardiac monitor and pulse oximetry. Automated BP cuffs or an arterial line are very useful for monitoring the patient's BP. A Foley catheter should be placed in the bladder, and a urine output of at least 30 to 50 mL/h (1 mL/kg per hour in children) should be maintained. All patients should have samples for blood and urine cultures obtained before parenteral antibiotics are administered. Any other potential sources of infection (such as sputum) also should be cultured.

Patients who do not respond to fluids need vasopressor support. We usually start with a continuous IV infusion of dopamine at a rate of 2 to 20 μg/kg per minute, titrating to a systolic BP > 90 mm Hg. At rates $<$ 5 μg/kg per minute, dopaminergic effects (renal and mesenteric vasodilatation) predominate; at levels > 10 μg/kg per minute, alpha sympathomimetic effects (vasoconstriction) predominate. Patients who are unresponsive to dopamine may require IV drips with either norepinephrine 0.5 to 30 μg/min or epinephrine 2 to 20 μg/min.

Parenteral antibiotics should be instituted as early as possible after pan-culturing the patient. The initial choice of antibiotics is variable and often institution-dependent. In the immunocompetent patient, cefotaxime 2 g IV is a good initial choice. A combination of ampicillin 2 g IV and gentamicin 1.5 mg/kg IV also may be given. IV drug abusers need coverage for staphylococcal species, which can be achieved with nafcillin 1 to 2 g IV. In the neutropenic or immunocompromised patient, a combination of gentamicin 1.5 mg/kg IV and an antipseudomonal drug such as piperacillin 3 g IV or ceftazidime 2 g IV should be given. Anaerobic coverage with either metronidazole 1 g IV or clindamycin 900 mg IV should be considered when an intra-abdominal source is likely. These patients are extremely ill and will need to be sent to the ICU. There, the patient should have a Swan-Ganz catheter placed for proper management of fluid needs and vasopressor agents.

HIV INFECTION

AIDS has developed into a worldwide epidemic, and no matter where you work you will encounter patients with this lethal disease. Try to find out what the patient's last CD4 cell count was (just ask the patient). This will help predict the patient's clinical course. Severe immunosuppression is rare before the CD4 count falls to < 500/mL. Thrush is seen with CD4 counts between 200 and 500. As the counts fall to < 200/mL, *P. carinii* pneumonia becomes common. Cytomegalovirus retinitis, CNS toxoplasmosis, and cryptococcal meningitis usually are seen when the CD4 count falls to < 100/mL. Patients with AIDS usually present with one of the following complaints: fever, cough and/or dyspnea, an altered mental status, and dehydration or generalized wasting.

Fever

When AIDS was first described, most patients with an HIV infection and a fever were admitted for extensive inpatient workup. With improvement in the management of opportunistic infections, many patients now are managed in the outpatient setting.

The workup of a patient with HIV infection and a fever usually should include the following:

- A thorough physical exam with particular emphasis on the degree of hydration, the lungs, and the neurologic exam
- Chest x-ray
- Pulse oximetry and/or ABGs
- CBC with manual differential
- Urinalysis and culture
- Blood cultures
- LP (in the presence of meningeal irritation or altered mental status)

The following are indications for admission of the patient with HIV infection and a fever:

- Severe dehydration not responsive to oral rehydration
- Hypoxemia
- A new infiltrate on the chest x-ray
- Evidence of meningitis or a space-occupying lesion on the head CT scan
- Neutropenia—an absolute neutrophil count (ANC) < 500 to 1000; calculate ANC as follows:

$$ANC = (\% \text{ granulocytes} + \% \text{ bands})$$
$$\times \text{ WBC count}$$

- Severe wasting and lack of a social support system

Shortness of Breath and a Cough

Respiratory complaints are common in patients with HIV infection. Causes include infections, neoplasms, and other idiopathic processes. Tuberculosis should always be considered present until proved otherwise; all necessary precautions should be taken, and the patient should be placed in respiratory isolation immediately. Patients with a cough or dyspnea should have a chest x-ray, ABG, and sputum collection for Gram's stain, culture, acid-fast bacterial stains, and culture for tuberculosis. Calculate the patient's A-a gradient (see Chapter 2). An increased A-a gradient can be one of the earliest signs of *P. carinii* pneumonia even without significant hypoxemia.

Indications for admission include hypoxemia and the presence of a new infiltrate on the chest x-ray. If you suspect tuberculosis, the patient should be admitted to an isolation bed until tuberculosis is ruled out or the patient is no longer infectious (usually after 2 weeks of antituberculous treatment).

Altered Mental Status

The workup of a patient with HIV infection should be similar to that of other patients with an acute alteration in mental status. In addition, although not immediately indicated, patients with HIV infection should have a head CT scan performed with IV contrast. A ring-enhancing lesion suggests toxoplasmosis or lymphoma. After excluding a space-occupying lesion and mass effect, an LP should be performed to exclude meningitis.

Dehydration and Wasting

Patients with dehydration and severe wasting who are not responding to oral rehydration may require admission for IV hydration, especially if they do not have adequate home care.

14

CHAPTER

Orthopedic Injuries and Swollen Joints

It is beyond the scope of this chapter to review in detail all the various specific orthopedic injuries and their treatment. Instead, we emphasize the general assessment and management of common orthopedic injuries. We review indications for obtaining x-rays and orthopedic consultation, and we briefly cover the use of splints. Finally, we discuss the assessment and differential diagnosis of swollen joints, with particular emphasis on recognizing the septic joint.

GENERAL PRINCIPLES

Orthopedic injuries commonly are associated with other more immediately life-threatening injuries such as head, chest, or abdominal injuries. Therefore, the general guidelines reviewed in Chapter 3 should be applied to all orthopedic injuries as well. Also, isolated orthopedic injuries may in themselves be a threat to life or to limb. A femoral fracture, for example, can cause 1 to 2 L of blood loss and hypovolemic shock.

Always begin with a rapid primary survey with assessment of the patient's ABCs. Do not let yourself be distracted by a dramatic or intensely painful orthopedic injury. Rapid resuscitation and stabilization should always precede orthopedic management.

FRACTURES

Fractures are the result of bony injury and may be open (contiguous soft tissue injury and exposure to the external environment) or closed, displaced or nondisplaced. Fractures are described in terms of the direction of the fracture line (horizontal, vertical, oblique, spiral) and the direction and degree of angulation (always in reference to the most distal fragment). When the fracture results in more than two fragments, it is called *comminuted*.

History

Include the following information in the patient's history:

- Mechanism of injury: cause, intensity, and direction of forces
- Time of injury
- Degree of resulting dysfunction (can the patient move the affected limb or ambulate?)
- History of prior injuries
- Initial treatment
- Presence of audible clicks, pops, or snaps at the time of the injury (in knee trauma, this suggests injury to the meniscus or anterior cruciate ligament)
- History of chronic illnesses, such as diabetes, renal disease, or metabolic diseases (e.g., Paget's disease)

Physical Examination

To avoid errors of omission, always begin your exam with a comprehensive neurovascular assessment of the limb involved in the injury. All pulses should be palpated and documented before you perform any manipulations. In the absence of a palpable pulse, a portable Doppler should be used to assess an audible pulse. Vascular assessment also should include evaluation of skin color, temperature, and capillary refill. The neurologic exam should include assessment of sensation (pin prick in the lower extremities, two-point discrimination in the upper extremities) and motor function. Table 14–1 describes nerve injuries often associated with some of the more common orthopedic injuries.

Signs of a fracture include deformity, crepitus, swelling, ecchymosis, point tenderness, and loss of function. Only gross deformity or crepitus are definitive signs of a fracture. Always assess the entire limb as well as the adjacent joints for associated injuries. The most commonly missed fracture is a second fracture. Active range of motion as well as the ability to ambulate should always be assessed. Passive range of motion should not be attempted until you exclude a fracture.

Indications for x-rays include:

- Definite crepitus or deformity
- Obvious dislocations
- Significant *point* tenderness or swelling
- Functional impairment, including inability to bear weight
- Highly suggestive mechanism of injury
- Neurovascular impairment

At least two x-ray views (preferably three) showing trabecular detail taken at right angles to each other are necessary for assessment of any bony injury. When x-raying long bones, the joint above

Table 14–1. NERVE INJURIES ASSOCIATED WITH ORTHOPEDIC INJURIES

ORTHOPEDIC INJURY	NERVE INJURED	SENSORY LOSS	MOTOR WEAKNESS
Shoulder dislocation	Axillary	Deltoid region	Shoulder abduction
Humeral shaft	Radial	Dorsal 1st webspace	Wrist extension
Elbow, supracondylar	Median	Tip of 2nd finger	Thumb apposition
Elbow, lateral epicondyle	Ulnar	Tip of 5th finger	Finger abduction
Hip dislocation	Sciatic	Lateral leg and foot	Knee flexion, foot and toe flexion and extension
Knee dislocation	Tibial	Plantar foot	Foot flexion
Fibular neck	Peroneal	Lateral leg, foot dorsum	Foot extension

and below should be included to rule out concomitant dislocations. Contralateral comparative views can be extremely helpful in difficult cases, especially in children.

SPRAINS AND STRAINS

A sprain is an injury to a *ligament* (connects bone to bone); a strain is an injury to a *tendon* (connects muscle to bone). Sprains and strains can result in significant functional impairment and should never be brushed off as "only" a sprain or a strain. Sprains and strains are classified according to the severity of injury:

- **First degree:** Microscopic tears of tendon or ligament fibers. This results in mild to moderate pain and swelling over the area of the tendon or ligament with no joint laxity and minimal functional impairment.
- **Second degree:** A partial tear of the tendon or ligament. This results in significant pain and swelling with moderate joint laxity and functional impairment.
- **Third degree:** Complete tear of the tendon or ligament that may result in minimal to significant pain and swelling, depending on whether bleeding is contained within an intact joint capsule. Significant joint instability and dysfunction are noted. Often, surgical repair is required.

INJURIES IN CHILDREN

In children, the developing growth plate is the most vulnerable element in the extremities,

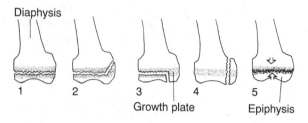

Figure 14–1. Schematic representation of the Salter-Harris classification of growth plate fractures.

whereas ligamentous or tendinous injury is unusual. Therefore with any painful injury to a bone you must rule out a growth plate fracture and treat as such.

Following is the Harris-Salter classification of epiphyseal injuries (Fig. 14–1) (use the mnemonic **M, E, ME,** to remember types II to IV):

- **Type I:** The fracture line runs through the growth plate. This often is impossible to identify on x-ray. Therefore, if there is significant tenderness over a growth plate, a type I fracture should always be assumed despite normal x-rays. Immobilize the involved limb and refer for orthopedic consultation, and repeat the x-ray in 10 to 14 days.
- **Type II:** The fracture involves the growth plate and the metaphysis (**M**). This is the most common growth plate fracture in children.
- **Type III:** The fracture involves the growth plate and the epiphysis (**E**).
- **Type IV:** The fracture involves the growth plate as well as both the metaphysis (**M**) and epiphysis (**E**).
- **Type V:** This is a compression fracture of the growth plate. This crush injury results in the greatest compromise to bony growth.

MANAGEMENT: GENERAL GUIDELINES

Reduction

Reduction of displaced fracture usually should be left to the orthopedist; in the presence of neurovascular compromise, however, you will be required to reduce the fracture. A grossly displaced fracture or dislocation should be placed in an anatomic position as soon as possible. Adequate sedation and analgesia usually is necessary and greatly facilitates reduction. Use of short-acting reversible agents such as fentanyl 1 to 2 µg/kg IV and midazolam 1 to 4 mg IV is recommended. Close monitoring of the patient and availability of antagonistic agents (naloxone 2 mg IV and flumazenil 1 to 3 mg IV), as well as airway management adjuncts, must be ensured before sedation.

Elements of reduction include:

1. Stabilization of the proximal fragment
2. Traction on the distal fragment along the long axis of the limb (often this alone will result in adequate reduction)
3. Reproduction of the forces that caused the initial injury
4. Reversal of the forces that caused the injury (this is why it is so important to try to understand the mechanism and forces that resulted in the injury)

Orthopedic Consultation

Urgent orthopedic consultation should be obtained in the following circumstances:

- Displaced fracture
- Neurovascular compromise

- Most fractures in children
- Open fractures
- Unstable fractures
- Fractures that require open reduction

Patients with open fractures should receive cefazolin 1 g IV or vancomycin 1 g IV as soon as possible after a sample from the wound is cultured. Tetanus prophylaxis should be considered (see Chapter 15).

Nondisplaced Fractures

You can remember how to manage nondisplaced fractures, as well as most sprains and strains, by using the mnemonic **RIICE:**

R=Rest

I =Ice—should be applied indirectly (have the patient wrap ice cubes in a plastic bag and cloth for 15 to 20 minutes every hour for the first 24 to 48 hours).

I =Immobilization—ED physicians should never apply circular casts, which can result in severe neurovascular dysfunction, especially as tissues swell. Preformed splints or those constructed from plaster of Paris or fiberglass should be used. (A more detailed description of splints will follow.)

C=Compression—achieved by using an elastic wrap (avoid vascular compromise).

E=Elevation—the involved limb should be elevated above the level of the heart to facilitate venous and lymphatic drainage, which will decrease pain and swelling.

All patients with fractures and third-degree sprains and strains should be referred to an orthopedic surgeon. Phone consultation with the surgeon before patient discharge is highly recommended.

SPECIFIC UPPER-EXTREMITY INJURIES

Although a comprehensive review of all fractures and dislocations is beyond the scope of this chapter, in this section we include several "pearls" of useful information for some of the more common injuries. For further information on the diagnosis and management of specific orthopedic injuries, refer to emergency medicine or orthopedic textbooks.

Shoulder Dislocations

Most dislocations are anterior; consider posterior dislocation in patients who have had a seizure or previous shoulder injuries. On exam, you will find flattening of the shoulder over the deltoid region, prominence of the acromion, or the ability to palpate the humeral head in the subcoracoid region. Neurovascular assessment should always be performed. Palpate the radial pulse, and assess pin-prick sensation over the deltoid region for evidence of axillary nerve injury (commonly associated with shoulder fracture dislocations).

Unless neurovascular compromise is present, obtain x-rays of the shoulder before reduction to exclude any associated fractures of the humeral head (particularly of the greater tuberosity) or of the surgical neck. The trans-scapular or "Y" view or the axillary view are particularly helpful in assessing the position of the humeral head in reference to the glenoid fossa. Sedation and analgesia (using a combination of a benzodiazepine and an opioid) usually are required to facilitate reduction. We like to place the patient prone and to apply increasing traction on the outstretched arm until reduction is achieved (Stimson's technique). Supe-

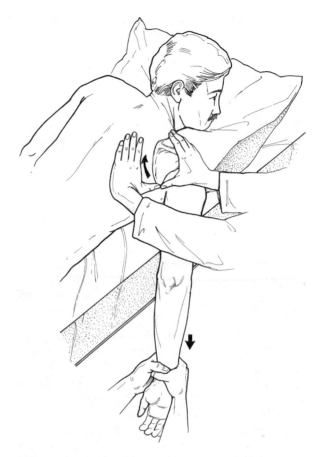

Figure 14–2. Shoulder reduction in the prone position. Traction is placed on the arm while the tip of the scapula is internally rotated by an assistant.

rior stabilization and internal rotation of the ipsilateral scapula often will help to reduce the shoulder (Fig. 14–2). The best results are achieved by relaxing the patient's musculature with midazolam 2 to 4 mg IV. After reduction, repeat films

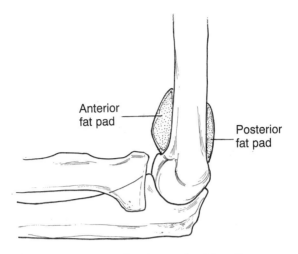

Figure 14–3. Lateral radiograph of the elbow region, demonstrating anterior and posterior fat pads.

should be obtained to ensure adequate reduction and to rule out fractures. The shoulder should be immobilized with an arm sling, and arrangements should be made for an orthopedic follow-up exam in 1 to 2 weeks.

Radial Head Fractures

The primary bony defect is difficult to see on routine x-rays. The presence of a posterior fat pad or bulging of the anterior fat pad (the "sail sign") on a lateral view of the elbow is diagnostic of a joint effusion and, in the presence of trauma, suggests a radial head fracture (Fig. 14–3). Aspiration of blood from the radiohumeral joint with injection of a long-acting local anesthetic is very effective in alleviating the associated pain and improving mobility. The arm should be put in a sling, allowing early mobilization in 3 to 5 days. Early physical therapy is key to achieving a mobile joint.

Supracondylar Fractures

Supracondylar fractures in children are very serious, especially if they are displaced. They can cause vascular compromise and often are difficult to reduce. Therefore, admission is necessary. Children with nondisplaced fractures can be sent home with a reliable adult, who must be taught to monitor for signs of vascular compromise, with the appropriate immobilization.

Scaphoid Fractures

Scaphoid fractures usually result from a fall onto an outstretched arm and hand. They often are not visualized on routine hand and wrist films, even after a scaphoid view is obtained. Because of poor blood supply, these fractures, especially if missed, can result in malunion or nonunion. When examining the patient, apply direct pressure to the anatomic snuff box. If tender, or if tenderness is elicited on axial compression of the thumb, suspect a scaphoid fracture and apply a thumb spica splint even if the x-ray is normal (Fig. 14–4). These injuries must be treated as though a fracture was seen on the x-ray. Orthopedic re-evaluation and repeat x-ray in 10 to 14 days is necessary.

Scaphoid Lunate Dislocations

To identify scaphoid lunate dislocations, look for widening of the space between the scaphoid and the lunate >3 to 5 mm (Terry Thomas' sign).

Perilunate/Lunate Dislocations of the Wrist

In these injuries, the third metacarpal, capitate, and lunate do not line up vertically on the lateral view of the wrist.

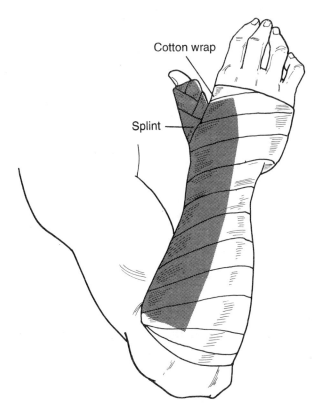

Figure 14–4. The thumb spica splint extending from the thumbnail to the mid forearm.

Boxer's Fractures

Fractures of the neck of the fifth metacarpal bone usually are secondary to the patient's punching a hard object. When the patient has punched someone in the face, you must suspect an associated human bite wound and look for a laceration. These often are deep, penetrating injuries due to the impact of the victim's teeth against the metacarpophalangeal joint. Admission for IV antibiotics and aggressive irrigation of the wound often are required. Gentle closing of the patient's fingers on the palm of your hand will demonstrate alignment of the metacarpal heads. Any angulation must be reduced. Boxer's fractures should be immobilized in an ulnar gutter splint. If there is >30° of volar angulation or significant rotational deformity, the patient should be referred to an orthopedist. Reduction of a third or fourth metacarpal fracture is very difficult and requires orthopedic intervention.

Bennett's Fracture

Bennett's fracture is a fracture of the base of the thumb metacarpal involving the joint. Adequate reduction usually requires surgery.

SPECIFIC LOWER-EXTREMITY INJURIES

Hip Fractures

Suspect a hip fracture when a patient, especially an elderly woman, presents with an unexplained fall. On exam, the injured lower limb may appear shortened and externally rotated. Early orthopedic consultation is required for all hip fractures. Always obtain appropriate films to rule out concomitant pelvic fractures in elderly victims of a fall. X-rays may not always reveal a fracture. All patients must be observed ambulating; any shuffling gait or abnormality suggests an occult fracture and requires that additional films be taken (e.g., a "frog's leg" Judet's view).

Hip Dislocations

Hip dislocations are most frequently posterior and often are associated with knee injuries because of the mechanism of injury (i.e., usually a force applied against the flexed knee with the hip in flexion). The leg usually is shortened and in internal rotation. Early reduction is necessary to avoid avascular necrosis of the femoral head. Injury to the sciatic nerve must always be excluded.

Knee Injuries

Any patient with a knee injury and significant pain or swelling or inability to bear weight requires knee films to exclude a fracture. A tense, painful, traumatic knee effusion should be evacuated. The presence of fatty globules in the joint indicates an intra-articular fracture (such as a tibial plateau fracture). Because knee injuries are accompanied by significant swelling, it often is difficult to diagnose specific ligamentous or meniscal injuries at the time of injury, and a complete knee evaluation may need to be done 5 to 7 days later when the swelling has decreased. Knee immobilization and crutches for ambulation should be given to patients with significant pain or inability to bear weight on the injured knee. A follow-up exam with an orthopedist within 1 week is recommended.

Patients with knee dislocations have a high incidence of accompanying popliteal arterial injury; thus, arteriography should be performed in these patients.

Ankle Sprains

In addition to examining the ankle for swelling, tenderness, deformity, and instability, palpate the fifth metatarsal as well as the *proximal* fibula for evidence of associated injuries. A complete neurovascular exam should always be included. Inability to bear weight, or direct tenderness over the tip or posterior aspect of the lateral or medial maleolus, requires a three-view ankle film series. The base of the fifth metatarsal should always be included in the film to rule out an avulsion fracture (traction by the peroneus brevis muscle) or a true Jones' fracture (a transverse fracture through the distal fibular diaphysis where both cortices appear thickened). X-ray of the foot is required when the patient has midfoot pain as well as inability to bear weight or tenderness over the navicular or fifth metatarsal.

SPLINTS

Splints, *not* circumferential casts, are the preferred method of immobilization in the ED. Splints can be useful in the following conditions: fractures, sprains, strains, joint infections, arthritis, tenosynovitis, lacerations that cross joints, deep space infections, and puncture wounds of the hands and feet. Rarely, if ever, is a circular cast indicated in the ED because of the potential for neurovascular compromise with swelling.

Plaster of Paris is a cloth impregnated with dextrose or starch and a semihydrated calcium sulfate. When water is added to the plaster of Paris, crystallization occurs, resulting in an exothermic reaction (which is more rapid and severe when hotter water is used, so use lukewarm water). Use between 8 and 12 layers of plaster. Cover the limb with stockinet to protect the skin; then wrap the limb with a single layer of soft cotton (Webril®) to create padding, which further protects the skin and bony prominences and allows for swelling.

Measurement of splint length should be made over the corresponding contralateral limb. Immerse the plaster of Paris in lukewarm water until all air bubbling ceases. Express excess water by wringing the plaster between your index and middle fingers. Apply the plaster to the affected limb, smoothing it out with the palms of your hands (the plaster should conform loosely to the limb). As the plaster hardens, apply a circumferential elastic wrap starting at the most distal level. Each wrap should overlap 50% of the prior wrap. Leave the distal end of the limb exposed to allow assessment of color and temperature. Fold back the end of the stockinet over the splint to create a smooth, padded edge. The plaster will harden within 15 to 30 minutes, but it continues to set for 24 hours, during which time weightbearing should be avoided.

SWOLLEN JOINTS

There are many causes of swollen joints, but in the absence of trauma, your main purpose is to identify patients with a septic joint. Staphylococcal, gonococcal, and pneumococcal organisms are the most common causes of septic arthritis and can rapidly destroy a joint if not quickly diagnosed and treated. If you can't rule out a septic joint, arthrocentesis must be performed.

History

In gathering information from the patient, ask the following questions:

- If multiple joints are involved, was there an additive or migratory pattern to the involvement?

- Are there associated symptoms such as a fever, chills, or rash?
- Is there any history of STDs?
- Is there any history of trauma?

Physical Examination

When performing the exam, ascertain the following:

- Is the joint hot, red, and swollen—or just swollen?
- Are there signs of generalized toxicity, such as fever, tachycardia, or hypotension?
- Are there signs associated with systemic lupus erythematosus, such as a malar rash, alopecia, or pharyngeal ulcers?

Gonococcal arthritis is suggested by the presence of discrete purplish papules over the extensor surfaces of the fingers, tenosynovitis, and/or a cervical or urethral discharge.

Laboratory Tests

The most important test is a joint aspiration, which must be performed in all patients with an atraumatic swollen joint in whom the possibility of septic arthritis is considered. Indications for arthrocentesis include:

- A solitary red or hot joint
- Monoarticular or oligoarticular involvement in the presence of fever or chills

Joint fluid should be obtained under strict sterile conditions and sent for CBC and differential, glucose, Gram's stain, crystals, and culture and sensitivity. Note that joint aspiration is contraindicated in the presence of overlying skin infection.

Table 14–2 classifies the various types of arthritis based on synovial fluid findings.

If septic arthritis is present, blood cultures as well as throat, cervical, urethral, and rectal cultures should be obtained. In the absence of septic arthritis, the following labs may be indicated: an ESR, an antinuclear antibody, a rheumatoid factor, an antistreptolysin titer, a Lyme titer, and a C-reactive protein.

Septic Arthritis

Patients with septic arthritis usually present with an abrupt onset of a red, hot, swollen joint. The most commonly involved joints are the knees, hips, and wrists. Often, these patients have associated fever and chills. Gonococcal arthritis, the most common cause of infection, often is associated with a periarticular tenosynovitis, particularly around the anatomic snuff box. As previously noted, typical skin lesions may be found.

If septic arthritis is a possibility, empirical IV antibiotics, such as cefotaxime 1 to 2 g IV, must be started as soon as joint and blood cultures are obtained. All patients with septic arthritis should be admitted to the orthopedic service.

Table 14-2. CLASSIFICATION OF ARTHRITIS BASED ON SYNOVIAL FLUID ANALYSIS

	NORMAL	NONINFLAMMATORY	INFLAMMATORY	SEPTIC	TRAUMATIC
Clarity	Transparent	Transparent	Transparent-opaque	Opaque	Opaque
Color	Clear	Yellow	Yellow-white	Yellow	Pink
Viscosity	High	Low	Low	Low	High
WBCs/mL	≤200	200–3000	3000–75,000	≥75,000	<200
%PMNs	<25	<25	>50	>75	<25
Glucose	= Serum	= Serum	<Serum	<Serum	= Serum

PMNs = polymorphonuclear leukocytes; WBCs = white blood cells.

15

Principles of Wound Management

Wounds are one of the most common problems encountered by emergency physicians. It is estimated that more than eleven million wounds are evaluated in EDs each year. The ultimate goals of wound management include restoration of function and optimal cosmetic results. Infection, which develops in 3% to 10% of wounds, adversely affects these goals. Therefore meticulous care should be given to minimize this complication.

HISTORY

The following information should be obtained:

- **When did the injury occur?** As more time elapses, the degree of bacterial contamination increases. When more than 10^6 bacteria are present in each 1 mL of tissue, infection is likely. It is commonly taught that if more than 6 to 12 hours have elapsed (the "golden period" of the wound), it is unwise to close the wound. In areas of good vasculature (e.g., face, scalp), however, the tissues' ability to resist infection is greater, and wounds can be closed up to 24 hours after the injury. Even in areas of good blood supply, however, if the wound appears highly contaminated, you should either excise the wound margins (thus creating a new wound if excess tissue is available) or defer wound closure for several days. (This is called delayed primary closure.)

- **What caused the injury?** Injury with a dirty, potentially contaminated object increases the likelihood of infection. Mammalian bites (e.g., dogs, cats, humans) increase the risk of infection.

- **Is there any possibility of retained foreign bodies?** Foreign bodies are present in approximately 3% of wounds and increase the risk of infection. Regular soft tissue x-rays, ultrasound, CT scanning, or even MRI can help identify a foreign body. All wounds should be probed manually for the presence of foreign bodies. (If sharp foreign bodies are likely, you should use an instrument to probe the wound.) Glass, the most common foreign body, usually is seen on regular x-rays regardless of its lead content. A skin marker and at least two views will help you determine where the foreign body is.

- **Was the wound cleaned after the injury?** What was used to clean the wound?

- **When did the patient last receive a tetanus shot?** Table 15–1 presents the current recommendations concerning the need for both active (tetanus immune globulin [TIG]) and passive (tetanus–diphtheria toxoid [Td]) tetanus prophylaxis.

- **Does the patient have any underlying immunocompromising conditions** (e.g., cancer, diabetes, steroid use, chemotherapy, AIDS)?

Table 15–1. RECOMMENDATIONS FOR TETANUS PROPHYLAXIS

	CLEAN MINOR WOUNDS		ALL OTHER WOUNDS	
History of tetanus immunization	Td	TIG	Td	TIG
Doses, uncertain to <3	Yes	No	Yes	Yes
Doses >3	No*	No	No†	No

*Yes, if more than 10 years since last dose.
†Yes, if more than 5 years since last dose.
Td = tetanus-diphtheria toxoid; TIG = tetanus immune globulin.

- **Is the patient allergic to antibiotics?** (This will affect your choice of antibiotics, if indicated.)
- **Is the patient allergic to local anesthetics?** (Ask if the patient has ever had local anesthesia given by a dentist.)

PHYSICAL EXAMINATION

Adequate examination and management of a wound usually requires local anesthesia. However, always perform and document a complete *neurovascular exam* before giving an anesthetic. Evaluate pulses and capillary refill distal to the injury. In the hand, two-point discrimination (using a paper clip bent in two) is the best sensory modality to be examined. Elsewhere, evaluate pin-prick sensation. Check range of motion to evaluate for tendon or ligament injury and muscle strength.

Table 15–2. CHARACTERISTICS OF
LIDOCAINE AND BUPIVACAINE

ANESTHETIC AGENT	ONSET	DURATION	ACCEPTABLE SAFE TOTAL DOSE
Lidocaine	2–5 min	30–120 min	4–5 mg/kg
Bupivacaine	5–10 min	4–8 h	2–3 mg/kg

WOUND PREPARATION

The cornerstone of management includes mechanical debridement of devitalized tissue and copious irrigation with a balanced physiologic solution such as NS.

Local Anesthesia

Local anesthetics (which stabilize cell membranes) are either esters or amides. An easy way to remember to which group a particular anesthetic belongs is to note that all amides have the letter "i" in their generic name before the suffix "caine" (e.g., lidocaine, mepivacaine). The importance of knowing the chemical class of a particular agent stems from the fact that most allergic reactions to local anesthetics are due to the esters or the methylparabate preservative used in lidocaine preparations. If a true allergy to lidocaine is present, you can use the parenteral form of diphenhydramine diluted 1:4 with NS as a local anesthetic.

The most commonly used local anesthetics are lidocaine and bupivacaine. Their onset, duration, and toxic ranges are presented in Table 15–2.

The addition of epinephrine to the local anesthetic causes vasoconstriction, resulting in improved hemostasis, decreased systemic absorption, and prolonged action. Epinephrine should be avoided in the digits, tip of nose, and tip of penis (think "nose, toes, fingers, hose").

To decrease the pain caused by infiltrating a local anesthetic, take the following steps:

- Use a small needle, preferably #27 gauge.
- Inject as slowly as possible.
- Dilute lidocaine 10:1 with sodium bicarbonate 8.5% IV solution (this diluted product has a shelf life of at least 1 week).
- Warm the local anesthetic to body temperature.
- Pinch the skin adjacent to the wound just before injecting the local anesthetic.
- Inject the local anesthetic into the SC plane instead of the intradermal plane (this has a longer onset but is much less painful).
- In clean wounds, insert the needle through the wound edges. (If the wound is contaminated, it is better to infiltrate the skin around the wound.) Enter at one end and slowly infiltrate the anesthetic around the wound in continuous circular advancements, so the patient will have to suffer only one needle stick (Fig 15–1).

Irrigation

Irrigation has been shown to be effective in removing both bacteria and infection-potentiating factors such as soil from the wound. The efficiency of irrigation is increased with higher pressures and volumes of fluid. We suggest irrigating with a 35- or 65-mL syringe with a #19-gauge angiocatheter. A minimum of 100 mL of crystalloid per 1 cm of wound should be used. If a large volume of irrigation is required, you can place a 1-liter bag of NS with attached IV tubing and a #18-gauge angio-

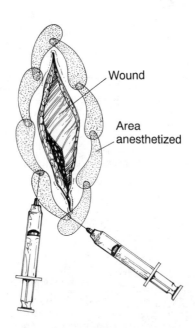

Figure 15–1. Anesthetizing the wound. The wound is anesthetized in a circular motion. With each successive injection, the needle enters a previously anesthetized area.

catheter at the end within a pressure cuff (those that are intended for rapid infusion of fluids). Maximally inflate the cuff and open the valve, which can be used to adjust the force of the stream through the angiocatheter. Pressures of 6–10 psi can be obtained and maintained throughout irrigation (Fig. 15–2). Commercially available transparent plastic shields that attach to the end of the syringe or IV tubing are useful for reducing splashing.

After adequate irrigation, the wound and its surrounding edges should be scrubbed with a dilute 1% povidone iodine solution (do not use the scrub solution intended for prepping operative fields in

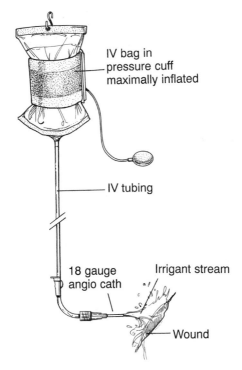

Figure 15–2. Simple set up for high pressure irrigation. The IV bag is placed within a fully inflated pressure cuff.

the operating room). Do not irrigate the wound with alcohol, hydrogen peroxide, or concentrated betadine solution.

Debridement

Devitalized, crushed, avascular tissue forms an excellent medium for bacterial growth; therefore, it is essential to remove as much devitalized tissue as possible. Adequate debridement sometimes re-

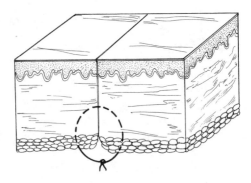

Figure 15–3. Deep suture. Note that the knot is buried in the depth of the wound.

quires the use of local flaps or grafts for closure of the remaining defect. In these cases, it probably is best to consult the plastic surgeon.

WOUND CLOSURE

Now you are ready to close the wound. Options for wound closure include:

1. **Sutures**—in general there are two types of sutures:
   a. *Absorbable sutures* are biodegradable (either by enzymatic degradation or phagocytosis) and cause more tissue reaction than nonabsorbable sutures. They are used mainly SC, but in children a rapidly absorbed suture can be used to avoid the need for suture removal. If the wound edges are not closely approximated before repair, use deep sutures to reduce the tension on the superficial sutures (Fig. 15–3). Vicryl usually lasts 6 to 8 weeks, during which time healing

re-establishes 70% of the wound's original tensile strength. Dexon is a good alternative. Chromic or catgut (which is absorbed within 2 to 3 weeks) can be used for repair of intraoral lesions.

b. *Nonabsorbable sutures* are used for skin closure and require removal. Choose a non-braided monofilament suture, which is easy to handle and causes minimal tissue reaction. Nylon is the most commonly used suture. Prolene, though slightly more expensive than nylon, is more pliable and easier to tie.

As the number of zeros decreases, there is an increase in the tensile strength of the suture, but greater tissue reactivity results. For the face, use a 5/0 or 6/0 suture. In the digits, a 5/0 suture should be used. Everywhere else, a 4/0 suture usually is adequate.

2. **Staples** can be placed rapidly with relatively little discomfort. They are especially useful in scalp lacerations not involving the galea, but they may be used anywhere on the body when you need to save time. Note that staples can cause artifacts on CT scans and are a poor method for achieving hemostasis.

3. **Steri-strips** are painless, do not require suture removal, and can be applied rapidly. Always use an adhesive such as tincture of benzoin or preferably Mastisol (Ferndale Laboratories, Ferndale, MI) around the wound to enhance adhesion. Avoid contact of the adhesive with the wound. In gaping or very deep wounds, or over areas of frequent motion and tension, Steri-strips should not be used.

4. **Biologic adhesives:** Histoacryl is an excellent alternative for superficial wounds anywhere on the body, but it is not yet FDA-approved in the USA.

Helpful Tips for Wound Closure

- Tie your knots just enough to approximate wound edges. Do not tie too tightly; this will only strangulate the tissues and cause necrosis and sloughing of the edges. (Remember that tissue swelling will increase during the next 24 to 48 hours.)
- Take equal "bites" from both sides of the wound. More tissue should be taken at the depth of the wound than at the surface (Fig. 15–4).
- Try to evert the wound edges. If you have difficulty doing this, use a vertical mattress suture (Fig. 15–5). Sometimes it is useful to alternate simple with mattress sutures to achieve eversion yet save time.
- If one side of the wound is longer than the other, use wider spaces between adjacent sutures on the longer side. This may avoid forming a "dog ear" at the end. The management of a dog ear is illustrated in Figure 15–6.
- The length of the suture ends should be roughly equal to the distance between adjacent sutures. Don't cut the sutures too close to the end. This will only make suture removal more difficult.
- Closure of scalp wounds can be facilitated by tying knots in the hair to keep wound edges together.

Wound Dressings

Most wounds should be covered with an antibiotic ointment such as bacitracin and a dry gauze or Band-Aid. In areas of hair, bacitracin alone is adequate. By the way, the purpose of shaving hair around the wound is to facilitate wound closure, not to reduce wound infection. In fact it may in-

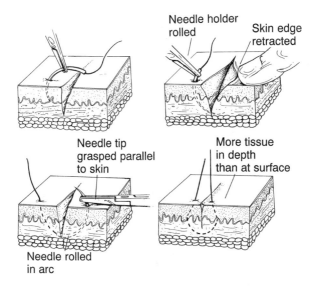

Figure 15–4. Placement of a simple suture. By holding the needle upside down and excessively pronating the wrist, the needle tip moves farther away from the laceration with deeper penetration. Thus there is more tissue at the depth of the wound, causing eversion of the wound.

crease the risk of wound infections. The use of hair clippers is preferred. **Never shave the hairs of the eyebrow.**

Suture Removal

The timing of suture removal usually can be determined by wound location:

- Face: 3 to 5 days
- Extremities and digits: 10 to 14 days
- Trunk: 10 days
- Elsewhere: 7 to 10 days

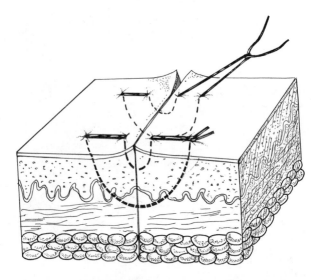

Figure 15–5. Vertical mattress sutures for approximation and eversion of skin edges.

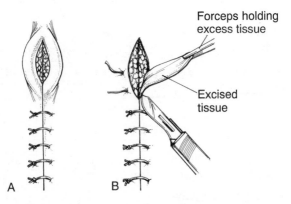

Figure 15–6. Correction of a "dog ear." *A*, Presence of a dog ear; *B*, excision of dog ear with closure of defect.

PATIENT INSTRUCTIONS FOR WOUND CARE

The following instructions should be given to all patients:

- Keep the wound clean and dry. After 24 to 48 hours, the wound may be washed gently and then covered with a clean dressing.
- If the wound is on an extremity, elevate the extremity for 48 hours to reduce swelling.
- Return to the ED if there is increasing swelling, redness, or pain around the wound; yellow or green discharge from the wound; fever; or shaking chills.

INDICATIONS FOR CALLING A PLASTIC SURGEON

Always let the patient (or his or her parents) know that a scar is unavoidable yet can always be corrected at a later date (usually after at least 6 to 12 months) if necessary. A plastic surgeon should be consulted in the following circumstances.

- When the wound involves the lacrimal apparatus or the canthal ligaments of the eye.
- When there is extensive tissue loss requiring grafting or complex local flaps other than simple undermining of the wound edges.
- When lacerations involve the corner of the mouth or the philtrum ("Cupid's bow").
- When the patient or family insists that you call a plastic surgeon.

ANTIBIOTICS

The use of antibiotics prophylactically is very controversial; it should never be a routine practice. The following are generally accepted indications for prophylactic use of antibiotics:

- **Human bites:** All patients with significant bites (i.e., *not* superficial abrasions) probably should receive antibiotic prophylaxis. Immunocompromised patients and patients whose lacerations are over the metacarpophalangeal joints (as the result of punching in the mouth) often require admission for IV antibiotics. Common infecting organisms include *S. aureus*, streptococci, anaerobic organisms, and *E. corrodens*. Give augmentin 500 mg PO tid, cefuroxime axetil 500 mg PO bid, or clindamycin 150 mg PO qid. Patients who are sent home should always return for a wound check within 24 to 48 hours.
- **Dog bites:** Always assess the possibility of rabies, which is more common in cases of unprovoked dog bites or bites by wild dogs. Infections usually are due to *Staphylococcus* species. *P. multocida* is less likely and a mixed flora is commonly involved. Antibiotic prophylaxis usually is not indicated except when there are extensive hand bites. Augmentin or a first-generation cephalosporin is a good choice.
- **Cat bites** result in infection 30% of the time, usualy due to *P. multocida* or *S. aureus*. Give augmentin or a first-generation cephalosporin (e.g., cephalexin 500 mg PO qid).
- **Rabies** is most likely to be present in cases of raccoon, bat, and skunk bites. It is unlikely in rodent bites. In cat or dog bites, ask about the immunization status of the pet. If the rabies

immunization status is unknown, suggest that the animal be observed by the owner for 10 days. Contact the local health department for suspicious bites. In cases of exposure to an animal suspected to have rabies, give human rabies immune globulin 20 U/kg (half around the wound, half IM) plus human diploid cell vaccine 1 mL IM immediately, then 1 mL IM on days 3, 7, 14, and 28. Rabies vaccine absorbed can also be given instead of the human diploid cell vaccine—1 mL IM immediately, then 1 mL IM on days 3, 7, 14, and 28.

- **Open fractures** should receive antibiotics. Give a first-generation cephalosporin or dicloxacillin 500 mg PO qid. Many patients with open fractures need to be admitted for operative repair and/or debridement. Always consult an orthopedic surgeon.

16

CHAPTER

Environmental Disorders

BURNS

Burns are the result of thermal injury and are caused by scalding fluids, steam, fire, electricity, or chemicals. In the past, fluid loss was a major cause of mortality; today, inhalational injury and sepsis are the major contributing factors. Therefore, in addition to aggressive fluid management, early recognition of inhalational injury and appropriate management are paramount. Remember too that the patient may also have other significant injuries, and should be managed as any other multiply injured patient.

The prognosis of burn victims depends on the patient's age, the extent of the burn (percentage of body surface area [% BSA]), the burn depth, the presence of associated inhalational injury, and the patient's past medical history. Therefore, every one of the above factors must be assessed.

History

Include the following information in the patient's history:

- What caused the injury?
- What kind of material was combusted?
- Did the injury occur in a closed space?
- Is there any evidence of inhalational injury?
- Was the patient conscious at the scene?
- What treatment was already given at the scene and en route (e.g., O_2, fluids)?
- Does the patient have any underlying medical illnesses or immunocompromising conditions?

Initial Assessment and Management of the Burn Victim

Airway

It is essential that you immediately determine whether there are any signs of present or impending airway compromise. Facial edema, singed nasal vibrisae, perioral burns, and carbonaceous sputum should all increase your degree of suspicion of inhalational injury. Laryngeal edema can develop extremely rapidly, making endotracheal intubation very difficult or impossible. Therefore, if there is any suggestion of airway compromise, intubate the patient early. Try to use a large endotracheal tube (at least an 8.0 mm ID) so that bronchoscopy can be performed through it. If there already is significant laryngeal edema making intubation impossible, you will need to perform a cricothyroidotomy.

Breathing

Inhalational injury secondary to toxic fumes or steam as well as CO or cyanide poisoning should always be suspected. All patients should receive 100% supplemental O_2 while ABGs and carboxyhemoglobin levels are being obtained. For a more detailed review of CO and Cn poisonings, see Chapter 10. Patients who fail to maintain adequate oxygenation ($Pao_2 < 60$ mmHg on 100% O_2) or ventilation ($Paco_2 > 50$ mmHg) require intubation and mechanical ventilation.

Circulation

Burns can cause significant external fluid loss as well as large internal fluid shifts. Rapidly assess the patient's hemodynamic stability based on his or her mental status, skin perfusion, vital signs, and urine output. Establish IV access with at least two large-bore IV catheters, preferably through intact skin (IVs can be placed through injured skin if no other sites are available). Femoral lines or saphenous venous cutdowns present a high risk for infection or thrombosis and should be avoided. Monitor urine output closely using an indwelling urethral Foley catheter.

Fluid Resuscitation

Most hospitals use lactated Ringer's solution. The patient's fluid requirements during the first 24 hours can be estimated with the Parkland formula: 2 to 4 mL/kg per % BSA (up to 50%) burned should be given during the first 24 hours (only second- and third-degree burns should be considered in calculating percentage of BSA). Half of the requirements should be given within the first 8 hours from the time of the injury (*not* from the time of presentation). Adjustments should be made based on clinical parameters such as vital signs, urine output, or central venous pressure.

Assessment of the Burn

Depth

Burns are classified according to depth:

- **First-degree burns** involve only the epidermis, causing erythema and pain.
- **Second-degree burns** involve the epidermis and part of the dermis, causing blistering and severe pain.
- **Third-degree burns** involve the epidermis and all elements of the dermis as well as subdermal tissues. (Involvement of muscle sometimes is referred to as fourth-degree burns.) Third-degree burns are characterized by coagulation of blood vessels and white, shiny, leathery skin. These burns do not blanch and usually are not painful because the nerves are destroyed.

Percentage of Body Surface Area

This can be estimated roughly by using the patient's palm, which equals 1% of the total BSA, as a reference. In adults, use the "rule of nines":

head = 9%
anterior trunk = 18%
posterior trunk = 18%
upper limb = 9%
anterior lower limb = 9%
posterior lower limb = 9%
genitalia = 1%

In children the head is larger and the lower limbs smaller in proportion to adults (Fig. 16–1).

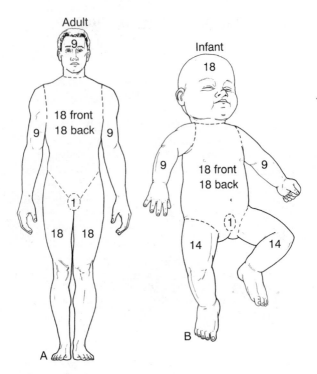

Figure 16–1. The Rule of nines for calculating the body surface area in an (*A*) adult and a (*B*) child.

Local Treatment of Burns

In third-degree burns, eschars (i.e., necrotic burned tissues) are stiff and, if circumferential, can compromise circulation (in the limbs) or breathing (in the trunk). If there is any evidence of compromise, perform an escharotomy using a #10 scalpel along the sides of the arms, legs, digits, or chest as required (Fig. 16–2). Anesthesia is not required, and the incision should be deep enough to allow the scar to expand and the SC fat to bulge, thus improving circulation or ventilation.

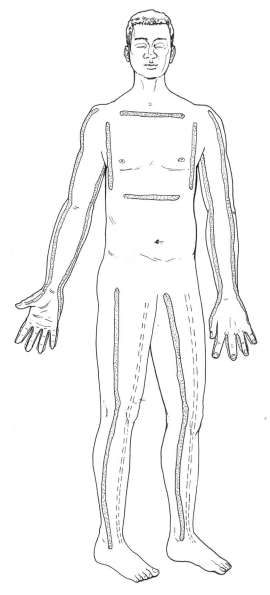

Figure 16–2. Performing escharotomies.

Cleanse second-degree burns with a balanced crystalloid solution (avoid cold fluids, which can cause hypothermia secondary to heat loss). Gently debride ruptured blisters. Then, cover the burns with a sterile dressing. If the patient is to be discharged, use an antimicrobial cream such as bacitracin or silver sulfadiazine.

Disposition

Indications for admission to the hospital include:

- Second-degree burns covering > 20% BSA in adults (> 15% in children)
- Third-degree burns covering > 10% BSA in adults (> 5% in children)
- Burns involving the hands, feet, eyes, ears, or perineum
- High-voltage electrical burns
- Significant underlying illnesses
- Extremes of age (infants < 1 year of age, elderly > 65 years)

Patients who are discharged should be instructed to elevate the involved limb (this will decrease swelling and pain) and to return to the hospital if there is any evidence of infection (fever, chills, pus, or increased redness). All wounds should be re-evaluated within 48 hours. Systemic antibiotic prophylaxis is not indicated. Tetanus prophylaxis should be given in accordance with the guidelines presented in Chapter 15.

COLD INJURIES

Hypothermia

Hypothermia is defined as a body temperature < 35°C and can result from multiple factors leading to increased heat loss, decreased heat production, or impaired thermogenesis due to central mechanisms. The most common cause of hypothermia is ambient exposure. The most common of the numerous predisposing conditions are alcohol ingestion, hypoglycemia, sepsis, hypothyroidism, and hypoadrenalism.

Hypothermia is classified by the degree of core temperature reduction:

1. **Mild hypothermia:** 32.5°C to 35°C
2. **Moderate hypothermia:** 27.5°C to 32.5°C
3. **Severe hypothermia:** < 27.5°C

The first response is shivering, which effectively generates heat by increasing the metabolic rate two to five times. As glycogen stores are depleted and the body temperature reaches 30°C, this response is also lost. The second response to cold exposure is vasoconstriction, which usually fails at temperatures below 24°C.

Alcohol ingestion often is a confounding factor because it increases heat loss by vasodilatation while altering a person's judgment as to the need to wear protective garments.

Hypothermia affects many systems:

- **Cardiovascular:** An initial tachycardia is followed by a progressive and severe bradycardia secondary to a decrease in the spontaneous firing rate of the cardiac pacemaker cells (this is why bradycardia secondary to hypothermia is usually refractory to standard treatment such as atropine). The most characteristic ECG abnormality in patients with hypothermia is the J-Wave (Osborn wave) or hypothermic hump (Fig. 16–3). Most commonly, this appears at temperatures < 25°C yet can be seen at temperatures < 32° C.
- **CNS:** Cerebral metabolism decreases approximately 6% to 7% for each degree of temperature change between 25°C and 35°C, and the

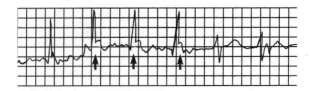

Figure 16–3. Hypothermic J waves.

EEG becomes flat at approximately 20°C. Deep tendon reflexes often are lost at temperatures < 30°C.

- **Renal:** Initially there is a diuresis, followed by a drop in renal blood flow.
- **Respiratory:** Respirations become slow and shallow.

Management

The most important factor in management of hypothermia is early recognition and rapid rewarming of the patient. Although detection of hypothermia is simple, the diagnosis often is missed in the ED. ED staff may fail to measure temperatures at all, especially in resuscitations (note: if a resuscitation effort is not succeeding, check the patient's core temperature). Additionally, be sure to check the temperature of all patients with an altered mental status or irrational behavior (especially the elderly). Another reason for missing hypothermia is the thermometer itself. Many thermometers, even electronic ones, fail to detect temperatures < 34.5°C. Always use special hypothermia thermometers. Rectal, esophageal, or tympanic probes can help estimate the core temperature.

Resuscitation should begin, as always, with assessment of the ABCs and the usual care of any patient with an altered mental status (see Chapter 7 for more details). Stabilization of the ABCs (with intubation and ventilation as required) and IV insertion should be followed by administration of glucose (as indicated by a Dextrostix), thiamine, and naloxone. If the patient is in ventricular fibrillation, an attempt should be made to defibrillate 3 times only, although antiarrhythmic drugs and electrical defibrillation rarely will be effective before the patient is warmed. Intubation should be performed as gently as possible, as it may theoretically induce ventricular fibrillation. A Foley catheter and gastric tube should be placed in most patients.

Blood samples should be obtained for toxicology screen, coagulation profile, creatinine phosphokinase (CPK), thyroid function tests, CBC, cortisol, and ABGs (measured ABG values rather than corrected values should be used for patient care).

Rewarming Methods

- **Passive external warming** consists of placing the patient in a warm environment, providing warm clothing, and allowing the body to regain heat. This treatment is limited to patients with *mild hypothermia.*
- **Active external rewarming** involves the external application of heat such as hot water bottles, warm blankets, or even immersion in a tub of warm water and is indicated for patients with *moderate hypothermia* when more advanced facilities are unavailable.
- **Active core rewarming** is the application of heat into the core or central parts of the body. Warmed inhaled oxygen is the simplest method. A 1-liter IV bag of crystalloids in fluid can be warmed in a microwave on high heat for 2 minutes; this brings the fluid to a temperature of approximately 38.2°C. Before administering, mix the fluid vigorously and check its temperature by placing a tempera-

ture probe in the middle of the bag. Esophageal or rectal lavage with warmed fluids also can be performed (avoid irrigating the area containing the temperature probe). More invasive methods include peritoneal lavage, pleural lavage, and cardiopulmonary bypass (either full or partial) using warmed fluids. Active core rewarming is appropriate for patients with severe hypothermia or those with hemodynamic impairment.

Remember that a patient should never be pronounced dead until *warm and dead*. All resuscitative efforts should be continued until the patient's core temperature reaches 32°C.

Frostbite

Frostbite is a form of local tissue injury due to freezing cold, whereas *trench foot* occurs with prolonged exposure to wet (yet nonfreezing) cold temperatures. The most commonly involved areas are those farthest from the body core with the poorest blood supply, such as the feet, hands, nose, earlobes, and cheeks. Predisposing factors include alcohol or other vasodilating drugs, malnutrition, anemia, poor local circulation, and cigarette smoking.

Frostbite is divided into superficial and deep injuries. In superficial frostbite, large clear blisters (resembling a second degree burn) appear, followed by hardening and darkening of the skin. However, beneath the surface, the skin remains soft and pliable. In deep frostbite, the tissues are deep purple or red and cool to the touch. Sensation and distal function are often absent and the tissues feel woody and stony.

Early prediction of the severity of injury is very difficult, and partial or full recovery may be the result of an initially necrotic-appearing limb. Therefore, any decisions concerning surgical treatment should be delayed until clear demarcation is apparent, approximately 6 months later.

Management

Wet or cold garments should be removed immediately. Excessive manipulation of frostbitten extremities should be avoided. Rapid rewarming of the frozen part is the most important measure. This can be achieved by immersing the injured tissue in 42°C circulating water until a distal flush of the extremity is noted. Dry heat can be very dangerous and should be avoided. Recently, aloe vera (a selective inhibitor of thromboxane A_2), together with an oral NSAID such as ibuprofen, has been suggested as an effective local treatment for frostbite. Hemorrhagic blisters should be left alone, but clear blisters probably should be debrided. Although systemic antibiotic prophylaxis is not indicated, local antibiotics such as bacitracin or silver sulfadiazine can be used. Involved extremities should be elevated, and cotton should be placed between the toes and fingers. Tetanus prophylaxis should be considered and administered as described in Chapter 15.

Indications for admission include:

- Concomitant hypothermia
- Severe underlying or immunocompromising diseases
- Significant facial involvement
- Bilateral extremity frostbite
- Frostbite involving most of one limb

HEAT INJURIES

Heat Stroke

Heat stroke is a condition characterized by failure of central thermoregulation; patients present with a high fever (usually defined as > 41°C) and an altered mental status. In the past it was believed that heat stroke always was associated with anhidrosis, but young patients with exertional heat stroke may present with diaphoresis.

Remember that the patient's temperature may have fallen spontaneously or because of cooling before arriving at the ED. Therefore, do not exclude a heat stroke based on the initial ED temperature reading. Also, it is very important to rule out other life-threatening causes of hyperthermia including sepsis, meningitis, stroke, brain tumors, head injuries, and withdrawal from substances of abuse. Be wary of heat strokes especially during hot, humid weather and in patients who collapse after extreme physical exertion.

History

In obtaining the patient's history, ask the following questions:

- Did the symptoms follow strenuous physical activity?
- Were the symptoms concurrent with headaches, stiff neck, or vomiting?
- Is there a history of any disorders that interfere with sweating and therefore heat loss (such as icthyosis, psoriasis, etc.)?

Assessment

Begin by assessing the ABCs. Patients with heat stroke who are unconscious or lethargic may need to be intubated to protect their airway. Patients with heat stroke often are dehydrated; establish IV access and start fluid resuscitaton as required. Check a Dextrostix and give $D_{50}W$ 50 mL IVP if the glucose level is low, as well as thiamine and naloxone, as you would for all patients with an altered mental status. Accurate measurement of the core temperature with a rectal, esophageal, or tympanic probe is necessary for early recognition and treatment. Examine the patient for evidence of an infectious disease, head injury, or stroke. Draw blood for CBC, Chem 7, PT, PTT, ABGs, CPK, and urinalysis. Myoglobinuria is common and should be treated with alkalization of the urine and forced diuresis. Disseminated intravascular coagulation (DIC) may occur and should be treated with coagulation factors (i.e., fresh frozen plasma) and platelet replacements as necessary.

Treatment

Cooling the patient forms the cornerstone of treatment. Undress the patient and start cooling as soon and as quickly as possible. Patients who are alert and hemodynamically stable can be placed in a tub filled with cold water or ice. If a tub is unavailable or the patient is not stable, spray him or her with water mist and place the patient under a high-speed fan. Aggressive cooling should be continued until the patient's temperature falls to < 38.5°C (note: avoid overshooting and causing hypothermia). Fluid and electrolyte imbalance should be corrected as the clinical condition warrants. All patients with heat stroke need to be admitted.

Heat Exhaustion

Patients with heat exhaustion present with dehydration, nausea and vomiting, muscle cramps, and sometimes confusion. Their temperature is only moderately elevated. IV replacement of fluid and salt depletion with a balanced isotonic solution usually is required. This condition often is seen in poorly acclimatized patients who exert themselves in hot, humid climates. If severely dehydrated, these patients must be admitted.

Heat Cramps

Heat cramps are caused by depletion of sodium caused by extreme physical exertion and sweating. Patients usually are afebrile and complain of muscle cramps. They should be treated with replacement of water and sodium losses, and most can be discharged. Patients should be encouraged to continue to consume large amounts of salt-enriched fluids at home, such as Gatorade or other mineral drinks.

NEAR DROWNING

Drowning is defined as death from suffocation after submersion in water, whereas *near drowning* refers to survival after submersion. *Delayed drowning* or *secondary drowning* occurs when a patient who was apparently doing well after surviving submersion suddenly deteriorates. Alcohol and drug abuse plays a significant role in many drowning and near drowning cases, especially among youths. In submersion accidents involving diving injuries, concomitant C-spine injuries are common and must be excluded. Myocardial ischemia, seizures, and hypothermia may also be factors in submersion accidents and should always be considered. In approximately 15% of cases, laryngospasm causes death due to asphyxia, referred to as "dry drowning."

In the past, much emphasis was put on differentiating between freshwater and saltwater drowning. In most cases, however, the quantity of aspiration is not large enough to cause significant electrolyte shifts or hemolysis; *hypoxemia* is the major cause of morbidity and mortality. Hypoxemia can result from surfactant washout (leading to atelectasis), ventilation-perfusion mismatch, or damage to the alveolar capillary membrane. Noncardiogenic pulmonary edema can result from direct pulmonary injury.

History

In obtaining the patient's history, ask the following questions:

- How long was the patient under water?
- What was the temperature of the water?
- Did the patient require resuscitation?
- How soon after submersion did resuscitation begin?
- Does the patient have any underlying diseases, such as ischemic heart disease, seizures, or diabetes?
- Was there any evidence of drug or alcohol ingestion before the accident?
- What type of water was involved (fresh or salt water)?

Management

Assessment of the patient's ABCs with C-spine precautions and immobilization should be performed as soon as the patient arrives at the ED. Always look for associated injuries or underlying causes. All patients will need supplemental O_2. Patients who are obtunded or who remain hypoxic ($Pao_2 < 60$) despite O_2 therapy must be intubated and mechanically ventilated. Some patients require PEEP to achieve adequate oxygenation. Hypotensive patients should receive aggressive fluid resuscitation, but central venous pressure monitoring may be required to avoid overhydration and pulmonary edema. Measure a rectal or esophageal temperature to rule out hypothermia, which may be either the cause or the result of the near drowning. The following labs should be obtained: C-spine, CBC, Chem 7, PT, PTT, urinalysis, ECG, ABGs, and a chest x-ray. Note that the CXR may or may not be helpful early on; often radiologic findings lag behind changes in the ABGs. A nasogastric tube should be placed to empty the stomach and to avoid any further aspiration. Placement of a urethral catheter will help monitor urinary output. Repeated boluses of sodium bicarbonate (1 mEq/kg IVP) should be given, as required, for metabolic acidosis (pH < 7.10). Antibiotics and steroids are not indicated. Arrhythmias, which often result from hypoxia and acidosis, should be treated with appropriate antiarrhythmics.

Indications for Admission

All patients who are hypoxemic and require O_2 must be admitted. Asymptomatic patients without evidence of significant submersion can be discharged. Asymptomatic patients who have had a significant submersion or mildly symptomatic patients should be observed in the ED for several hours and can be discharged if their chest x-ray and oxygenation level remain normal.

17

CHAPTER

The Difficult Patient

The "difficult patient" arouses feelings of animosity and hostility in the health care provider. Such patients include those who are verbally or physically abusive, intoxicated, suicidal, homeless, malodorous, and self-abusive. Often these negative feelings are aroused in the health care provider before he or she meets the patient, based on the nurse's report or the patient's chief complaint, or upon entering the patient's room. However, these patients are the ones who need your attention most. Remember that the patient's abnormal behavior may be the result of a serious underlying disease. Also, because of their social isolation, these patients are at risk for developing many serious illnesses. Therefore a thorough evaluation is always required. The somnolent alcoholic patient lying in your ED may simply be drunk, yet also might be suffering from a subdural hematoma, hypoglycemia, or a brain abscess.

THE VIOLENT PATIENT

It is always best to try to identify potentially violent patients before they actually become violent. The following are conditions when violent behavior should be anticipated:

- Alcohol or drug abuse
- Acute psychotic or manic disorder
- History of violent behavior
- Antisocial personality
- Severe psychomotor agitation (e.g., pacing, yelling)
- Patient already restrained or brought in by police

An actively violent patient must be restrained for his or her own protection from serious injury, as well as for the protection of the health care providers. Carefully document in the patient's chart why the restraint was necessary. Restraining the patient also will facilitate patient evaluation, which might otherwise be impossible. Never turn your back on or stay alone in a closed room with a potentially violent patient. Leave the door open and do not stand in the way if the patient should attempt to bolt out of the room. Also, you should always leave yourself an easy avenue of exit. Some patients, if placed in a quiet environment, can be "talked down." In other instances, a "show of force" is enough to subdue a potentially violent patient.

Enter the room with security and explain to the patient in a strong, steady tone that you are there to help. If the patient refuses to stay calm, tell him or her that you will need to use a restraint. Usually at least five people will be required to physically restrain a violent patient. Each member of the team should be assigned one limb, and the patient should be approached by all members simultaneously. The patient should then be put into a strong, four-point restraint and a posey (a thick cloth device intended to restrain the trunk). Placing the patient prone is usually more effective and safer in case of vomiting, but it makes the examination more difficult (Fig. 17–1). Explain to the patient that you are using a restraint to avoid further injury to anyone. All violent and suicidal patients

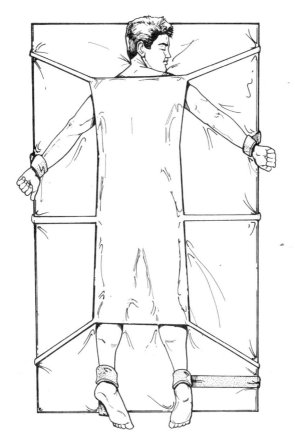

Figure 17–1. Physical restraint of a violent patient.

should be searched for weapons (which may be concealed in their undergarments).

Chemical Restraints

Physical restraints usually are sufficient, but often the violent patient requires a chemical restraint as well, such as a major (neuroleptics) or minor (benzodiazepines) tranquilizer. This protects the patient from injuries due to struggling against the restraint (e.g., rhabdomyolysis) and can facilitate evaluation.

Neuroleptics are particularly effective, having relatively few side effects such as cardiorespiratory depression. Haloperidol 5 mg IV or IM every 10 to 20 minutes is used most commonly. Note that IV use of haloperidol is not yet approved by the FDA. Droperidol, which has a more rapid onset and fewer adverse reactions, also can be given in doses of 2.5 mg IV or IM every 10 minutes. All neuroleptics can cause an acute dystonic reaction, which should be managed with diphenhydramine 50 mg IV or benztropine 2 mg IV.

Benzodiazepines can cause respiratory depression, yet are safer to use when seizures are a possibility (e.g., alcohol withdrawal, antidepressants, cocaine abuse). Lorazepam 1 mg IV or IM every 5 to 10 minutes or midazolam 0.5 to 1.0 mg IV can be given as needed. If you choose benzodiazepines, you should be prepared to intubate the patient if necessary. Use a cardiac monitor and pulse oximetry to monitor the patient. Frequent reassessment of the patient is required.

Differential Diagnosis

The differential diagnosis of violent behavior includes:

- Head trauma
- CNS infections
- Temporal lobe epilepsy
- Toxic substances (especially PCP, cocaine, ethanol)
- Withdrawal from substances of abuse
- Metabolic disorders (acute renal or hepatic failure)
- Psychiatric disorders: bipolar affective dis-

order (manic phase), schizophrenia (usually paranoid), and antisocial personality

Workup

Extensive workup of the violent patient usually is indicated in the following instances:

- Age extremes (> 50 or < 20 years old)
- Abnormal vital signs
- Abnormal physical findings
- No prior psychiatric history

The following tests should be considered in the workup: CBC, electrolytes, renal function tests, liver function tests, osmolarity, CT scan of the head, LP (especially if the patient has fever or signs of meningeal irritation), ethanol level, urine toxicology screen, and/or blood toxicology.

After underlying medical conditions are ruled out, violent patients should be seen by a psychiatrist.

THE INTOXICATED PATIENT

An alcoholic patient presenting with an altered mental status may be suffering from any of the following conditions:

- Acute intoxication with ethanol or mixed substances such as methanol, ethylene glycol, and/or cocaine
- Subdural hematoma or any other intracranial structural lesion
- Hypoglycemia, ketoacidosis, or electrolyte imbalance
- CNS infection
- Thiamine deficiency with acute Wernicke's encephalopathy

- Delirium tremens
- Any other medical problem unrelated to intoxication

All known alcoholic patients or patients with alcohol on their breath who present with an altered mental status should undergo a thorough physical examination to rule out any significant underlying diseases. Ascertain the following:

- Is there evidence of trauma?
- Is there nuchal rigidity?
- Is the patient febrile?
- Are there focal neurologic findings or signs of increased ICP?
- Were there any focal or new-onset seizures?

All intoxicated patients should have a rapid glucose determination by a Dextrostix, and consider obtaining a blood alcohol level. Most patients with an altered mental status should receive thiamine 100 mg IVP, $D_{50}W$ 50 mL IV (if their glucose is low or unmeasurable), and naloxone 2 mg IV as indicated. Continue to reassess these patients every 15 to 30 minutes for signs of deterioration. If the patient's blood alcohol level is not high, you should immediately proceed with an extensive workup for an altered mental status including blood labs, head CT, toxicology screen, and possibly an LP (see Chapter 4).

Indications for an urgent head CT in alcohol-dependent patients include:

- Focal or new-onset seizures
- Evidence of head trauma
- Signs of increased ICP or focal neurologic findings on exam
- An unimproved or deteriorating level of consciousness

If the initial alcohol level is high and the patient's level of consciousness improves, usually no further workup is necessary. As a rough estimate, non–alcohol-dependent patients metabolize alcohol at a rate of 15 to 20 mg/dL per hour. In alcohol-dependent patients the metabolism is enhanced, and the clearance increases to 25 to 30 mg/dL per hour. Remember that alcohol-dependent patients may have very high blood alcohol levels while acting completely sober.

THE HOMELESS PATIENT

Because of poor nutrition and hygiene, inaccessible medical care, and lack of social supports, otherwise benign illnesses can develop a malignant course among the homeless. Also, these patients tend to present for treatment much later in the course of their disease and therefore usually have a more serious illness. Soft tissue infections, pneumonia, and dehydration (which might otherwise be managed outside the hospital) often require inpatient care because of poor patient compliance and lack of stable medical follow-up.

Lack of adequate shelter exposes the homeless to the extreme elements and their associated conditions, such as frostbite, trench foot, hypothermia, heat exhaustion, and heat stroke. Therefore, a rectal temperature should be measured, especially during the cold months. Other commonly encountered problems in the homeless include malnutrition, skin ulcers, lice, scabies, alcohol abuse, trauma, viral hepatitis, tuberculosis, and mental illnesses.

If the patient is being discharged, a follow-up should be arranged. We recommend that you utilize social services in helping to arrange for proper disposition. If no alternative care is possible, have the patient come back to the ED for a follow-up.

18

Social and Legal Issues in the Emergency Department

Although an exhaustive (and exhausting) treatise on medical ethics and legal medicine is beyond the scope of this chapter, it will help you to have some familiarity with basic legal and ethical principles. For all of these issues, be sure to discuss problems with the attending physician, as the laws and protocols will vary from place to place. In this chapter we cover three issues: patient consent and leaving against medical advice, DNR orders and living wills, and domestic violence and rape.

CONSENT AND COMPETENCE

Two of the major guiding principles of medical ethics are *beneficence* (helping, or at least not harming, the patient) and *autonomy* (the right of every mentally competent adult to control his or her body). Autonomy requires that we obtain consent from a person to examine and treat them. Usually this is not a problem; occasionally, however, a patient will refuse treatment, forcing us into a conflict between beneficence and autonomy. Specifically, we have to decide whether we can treat this person against his or her will. To examine this a little more closely, it is useful to look at the types of consent we usually obtain for treatment.

Express consent means that a person specifically agrees to a particular examination or procedure. Legally this must be *informed consent* as well, meaning that the person has had the risks and benefits of the action, and alternative actions, explained before giving consent. Depending on your local protocols, this type of consent, often on a written form, may be required for certain procedures or treatments. *Implied consent* is the situation where a person, by his or her actions, can be assumed to have given consent (e.g., rolling up his or her sleeve when told that blood needs to be drawn). The doctrine of *emergency consent* is frequently encountered in the ED; it covers the situation where the patient is unable to give consent but requires life-saving treatment. The standard is to assume that the patient would consent in that situation to those procedures that a "reasonable person" would consent to.

The giving of consent assumes a competent, adult patient. The legal and ethical principles of autonomy hold that such a patient can refuse any examination or treatment. (Note that competency is a legal definition, ruled on by a judge. Physicians, including psychiatrists, cannot truly define someone as competent or incompetent to make decisions, although this is routinely and quite necessarily done in practice. What is actually being assessed, as termed by the legal system, is the "capacity" to make judgments.) Consent for a minor must be given by a competent adult who is the legal guardian. Note that this is not always the parent! If consent is not immediately available for a minor, the prevailing standard is for the physician to carry out care that is necessary to preserve life or limb, or to prevent the patient's condition from worsening. The problems that arise if a minor's guardian actually refuses to consent to a procedure which the physician deems necessary are beyond the scope of this chapter. If such a situation arises, discuss it with the attending physician.

As noted above, competent adults are able to refuse any treatment. If such a person does wish to leave the ED, he or she must be permitted to go. The great problem is defining who is competent. Sometimes this is obvious, as for example the patient with head trauma who doesn't even realize he's in the hospital. But what about the corporate vice-president with an acute MI who wants to leave now to go to an important meeting? In general, these people must be alert; oriented to self, time, and place; and must demonstrate that they understand the risks of leaving. The patient must not have any psychiatric disease that would impair judgment; most especially, he or she must not be suicidal. Document in the chart that you have explained these risks; be specific about what they are. Have the patient, and preferably an accompanying person such as a spouse, sign that note or an Against Medical Advice (AMA) form, if one exists at your institution. Sometimes a patient will refuse to sign anything. In this, case be especially sure that this person is competent by your assessment, document extremely thoroughly, and have someone sign the note as a witness to the patient's refusal to sign. Above all, whenever an "AMA situation" seems likely to arise, notify the attending physician.

LIVING WILLS AND "DO NOT RESUSCITATE" ORDERS

Patient autonomy can continue even after a person is no longer competent to give or refuse consent, if proper legal methods have been followed. Some examples of this are living wills and DNR orders. These occasionally can become extremely relevant in the ED setting. In general, what these instruments do is legally limit the types of care to be given to the patient. Be aware that a DNR order means just that: "Do Not Resuscitate." That means, in general, not to attempt any interventions if the patient is pulseless. It does *not* mean to withhold antibiotics, food, or even pressor agents in some cases. The DNR order also may not apply to certain circumstances, such as after a suicide attempt. The living will generally is broader in nature; often it will discuss the patient's desires about specific therapies. It also often names a health care proxy, a person who is legally assigned to make health care decisions for the patient. Be sure to involve such people in the decision process as soon as practical. A note of caution: If you have any doubt about a patient's supposed wishes, such as if you have only a companion's verbal statement that a person is a DNR, you are ethically and legally obligated to treat that patient as most people would wish to be treated (i.e., resuscitate). While this may result in the resuscitation of a person who did not wish that, such an action is far better than allowing a patient to die who would have wanted the resuscitation attempt to be made. Note that a patient can revoke a DNR order at any time merely by saying so.

RAPE, ASSAULT, AND ABUSE

A difficult legal issue that often arises is the intersection of the ED with the criminal justice system. Often the physician is bound by specific legal requirements. Specific situations that arise are rape, assault, and suspected child or elder abuse.

Always notify the attending physician when one of these situations arises.

Rape is a violent and traumatic crime. Initial evaluation must be directed to the patient's physical well-being. Injuries must be treated as they would for any other patient. As best as possible, of course, approach the patient in a nonthreatening and reassuring manner. Always have an observer/assistant present who is of the same sex as the victim. Once immediate physical problems are dealt with, you should get a brief history of the attack. Document physical findings appropriately on the chart, with particular attention to bruises and marks. Use a body map to describe the bruise. Obtain permission and take photographs of any marks or bruises, especially if the patient hasn't involved the police yet. Ask the patient if he or she wishes to involve the police. Get a rape crisis worker in to talk to the patient right away. The physical examination is facilitated by using a rape evidence kit. Follow local protocols for its use. The patient should receive treatment for STDs (usually IM ceftriaxone and oral doxycycline) and post-coital contraception if necessary (Ovral, two pills now and two in 12 hours). Appropriate referral for counseling and follow-up must be made.

In the case of a victim of assault, again the medical care of the patient is paramount. Because of the legal issues, the H&P exam should be documented meticulously. As with rape cases, ascertain if the victim wants the police to be involved, and make any such arrangements. Certain states require EDs to report felony assaults (e.g., gunshot wounds, knife wounds). Patients should be referred for counseling as well.

In the ED, you should always maintain a high degree of suspicion of abuse. All ages are susceptible to being abused, although children, women, and the elderly are more likely to be victims. As always, medical care is paramount. Whenever you do suspect abuse, you should notify the appropriate agencies; this usually is a legal requirement for physicians. Often, if not always, the hospital's social work department should be involved. Suspect abuse in the following situations:

- If a patient's injuries are inconsistent with the reported mechanism
- If a child's or elderly person's caregiver seems inappropriately unconcerned
- If the history given by the patient or caregiver is confused or changes markedly
- If the caregiver delays in bringing the patient for care

No one is "the wrong kind of person" to be an abuser; keep an open mind and a high degree of suspicion. When in doubt, it is totally appropriate to admit a patient while an investigation commences. Don't ignore your doubts.

Many resources exist to help you deal with the legal, social, and ethical difficulties that crop up in the ED. Clergy often are on call for patients who need or request them. They can help a family to deal with the stress of a death or serious illness, or to face decisions such as DNR status. The social work service of your hospital may have a full-time or on-call social worker; this person should be involved in all cases of possible abuse or neglect, and can be an additional support for families facing the stress of illness. Consider them also for patients with primarily social problems, such as the homeless, or for patients who may have psychosocial difficulties in addition to their medical problems, such as the elderly, patients with substance abuse problems, or patients who are having financial trouble that may compromise their care (e.g., preventing them from filling prescriptions.) Keep in mind that you are not alone, and use the help available to you.

THE DEATH OF A PATIENT

One of the hardest psychosocial situations you will face in the ED is informing a family of a patient's death, especially the death of a child. In general, you should have the family members placed in a separate and quiet room, preferably with a phone available. Have someone go in with you, such as a nurse, social worker, or member of the clergy. Usually the attending physician should be with you as well for at least part of the discussion. Be direct but supportive. Use the word "dead"; euphemisms such as "passed away" or "didn't make it" may not the get the message across. Always tell the family that you did everything you could. If possible, assure them that the death was painless and that their relative didn't suffer. After you have told them, stay in the room as long as needed to answer their questions. If the family is not present, it usually is best not to tell them over the phone. Instead, tell them that their relative is critically ill and that they ought to come in. Tell them to drive safely, and make sure they know how to get to the hospital.

Depending on the laws and procedures in your hospital, you may have to bring up the subjects of autopsy and organ donation to the family of the deceased. This can be very difficult, but it often is helpful to explain that such procedures allow the deceased to help others; for autopsy, point out that the information obtained may answer the family's questions about the cause of death, and provide useful medical information for relatives about inherited diseases (including cardiovascular disease). After you leave, someone should remain with the family to help them make funeral arrangements and inform other family members. Note that some deaths, varying from place to place, fall under the jurisdiction of the medical examiner or coroner. In these cases, you may be required to contact that official, and the family then must be informed that their relative is legally required to undergo an autopsy. Finally, remember to deal with your own feelings about the death. Don't hesitate to talk to co-workers, friends, or counselors if you are troubled.

TAKING CARE OF YOURSELF

A final note: throughout your work in the ED, keep yourself healthy. Get as much sleep as possible, eat appropriately, exercise regularly, and maintain your friendships and family relationships. Avoid alcohol, tobacco, or other harmful substances. Take care of yourself properly so you can take care of others properly.

Appendix A: Advanced Cardiac Life Support Algorithms*

---

*From Journal of the American Medical Association (1992;268:2171–2241), with permission, 1992, American Medical Association.

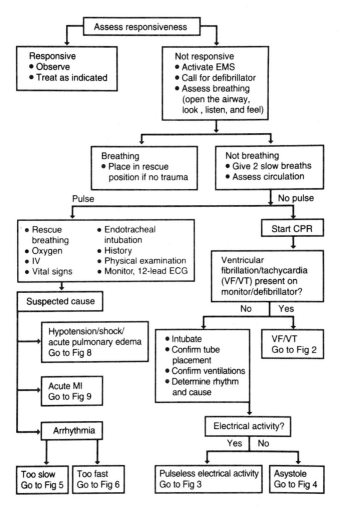

Figure 1. Universal algorithm for adult emergency cardiac care.

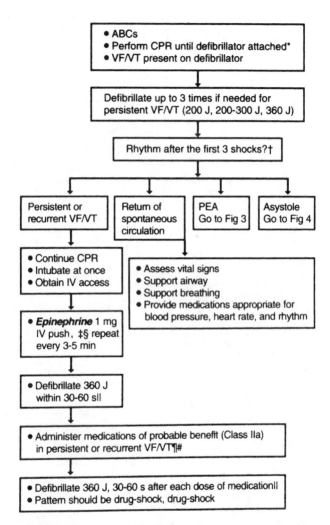

Figure 2. Ventricular fibrillation/pulseless ventricular tachycardia algorithm.

Class I: definitely helpful
Class IIa: acceptable, probably helpful
Class IIb: acceptable, possibly helpful
Class III: not indicated, may be harmful
*Precordial thump is a Class IIb action in witnessed arrest, no pulse, and no defibrillator immediately available.
†Hypothermic cardiac arrest is treated differently after this point. See section on hypothermia.
‡The recommended dose of *epinephrine* is 1 mg IV push every 3-5 min. If this approach fails, several Class IIb dosing regimens can be considered:
- Intermediate: *epinephrine* 2-5 mg IV push, every 3-5 min
- Escalating: *epinephrine* 1 mg-3 mg-5 mg IV push (3 min apart)
- High: *epinephrine* 0.1 mg/kg IV push, every 3-5 min

§ *Sodium bicarbonate* (1 mEq/kg) is Class I if patient has known preexisting hyperkalemia

‖Multiple sequenced shocks (200J, 200-300J, 360 J) are acceptable here (Class I), especially when medications are delayed

¶ • *Lidocaine* 1.5 mg/kg IV push. Repeat in 3-5 min to total loading dose of 3 mg/kg; then use
- *Bretylium* 5 mg/kg IV push. Repeat in 5 min at 10 mg/kg
- *Magnesium sulfate* 1-2 g IV in torsades de pointes or suspected hypomagnesemic state or severe refractory VF
- *Procainamide* 30 mg/min in refractory VF (maximum total 17 mg/kg)

• *Sodium bicarbonate* (1 mEq/kg IV):
Class IIa
- if known preexisting bicarbonate-responsive acidosis
- if overdose with tricyclic antidepressants
- to alkalinize the urine in drug overdoses
Class IIb
- if intubated and continued long arrest interval
- upon return of spontaneous circulation after long arrest interval
Class III
- hypoxic lactic acidosis

Figure 2. *Continued.*

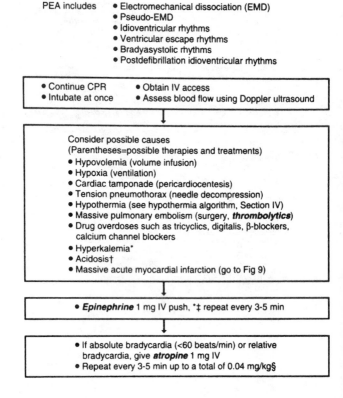

PEA includes
- Electromechanical dissociation (EMD)
- Pseudo-EMD
- Idioventricular rhythms
- Ventricular escape rhythms
- Bradyasystolic rhythms
- Postdefibrillation idioventricular rhythms

- Continue CPR
- Intubate at once
- Obtain IV access
- Assess blood flow using Doppler ultrasound

Consider possible causes
(Parentheses=possible therapies and treatments)
- Hypovolemia (volume infusion)
- Hypoxia (ventilation)
- Cardiac tamponade (pericardiocentesis)
- Tension pneumothorax (needle decompression)
- Hypothermia (see hypothermia algorithm, Section IV)
- Massive pulmonary embolism (surgery, *thrombolytics*)
- Drug overdoses such as tricyclics, digitalis, β-blockers, calcium channel blockers
- Hyperkalemia*
- Acidosis†
- Massive acute myocardial infarction (go to Fig 9)

- *Epinephrine* 1 mg IV push, *‡ repeat every 3-5 min

- If absolute bradycardia (<60 beats/min) or relative bradycardia, give *atropine* 1 mg IV
- Repeat every 3-5 min up to a total of 0.04 mg/kg§

Figure 3. Pulseless electrical activity algorithm.

Class I: definitely helpful
Class IIa: acceptable, probably helpful
Class IIb: acceptable, possibly helpful
Class III: not indicated, may be harmful

*$Sodium$ $bicarbonate$ 1 mEq/kg is Class I if patient has known preexisting hyperkalemia.

†$Sodium$ $bicarbonate$ 1 mEq/kg:

Class IIa
- if known preexisting bicarbonate-responsive acidosis
- if overdose with tricyclic antidepressants
- to alkalinize the urine in drug overdoses

Class IIb
- if intubated and long arrest interval
- upon return of spontaneous circulation after long arrest interval

Class III
- hypoxic lactic acidosis

‡The recommended dose of $epinephrine$ is 1 mg IV push every 3-5 min. If this approach fails, several Class IIb dosing regimens can be considered.
- Intermediate: $epinephrine$ 2-5 mg IV push, every 3-5 min
- Escalating: $epinephrine$ 1 mg-3 mg-5 mg IV push (3 min apart)
- High: $epinephrine$ 0.1 mg/kg IV push, every 3-5 min

§ Shorter $atropine$ dosing intervals are possibly helpful in cardiac arrest (Class IIb).

Figure 3. *Continued.*

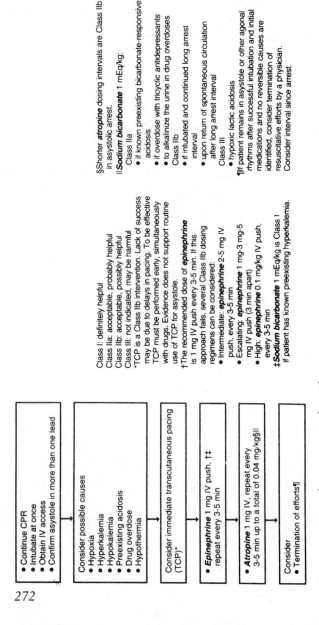

- Continue CPR
- Intubate at once
- Obtain IV access
- Confirm asystole in more than one lead

↓

Consider possible causes
- Hypoxia
- Hyperkalemia
- Hypokalemia
- Preexisting acidosis
- Drug overdose
- Hypothermia

↓

Consider immediate transcutaneous pacing (TCP)*

↓

- *Epinephrine* 1 mg IV push,†‡ repeat every 3-5 min

↓

- *Atropine* 1 mg IV, repeat every 3-5 min up to a total of 0.04 mg/kg§‖

↓

Consider
- Termination of efforts¶

Class I: definitely helpful
Class IIa: acceptable, probably helpful
Class IIb: acceptable, possibly helpful
Class III: not indicated, may be harmful

*TCP is a Class IIb intervention. Lack of success may be due to delays in pacing. To be effective TCP must be performed early, simultaneously with drugs. Evidence does not support routine use of TCP for asystole.

†The recommended dose of *epinephrine* is 1 mg IV push every 3-5 min. If this approach fails, several Class IIb dosing regimens can be considered:
- Intermediate: *epinephrine* 2-5 mg IV push, every 3-5 min
- Escalating: *epinephrine* 1 mg-3 mg-5 mg IV push (3 min apart)
- High: *epinephrine* 0.1 mg/kg IV push, every 3-5 min

‡*Sodium bicarbonate* 1 mEq/kg is Class I if patient has known preexisting hyperkalemia.

§Shorter *atropine* dosing intervals are Class IIb in asystolic arrest.

‖*Sodium bicarbonate* 1 mEq/kg:
Class IIa
- if known preexisting bicarbonate-responsive acidosis
- if overdose with tricyclic antidepressants
- to alkalinize the urine in drug overdoses
Class IIb
- if intubated and continued long arrest interval
- upon return of spontaneous circulation after long arrest interval
Class III
- hypoxic lactic acidosis

¶If patient remains in asystole or other agonal rhythms after successful intubation and initial medications and no reversible causes are identified, consider termination of resuscitative efforts by a physician. Consider interval since arrest.

Figure 4. Asystole treatment algorithm.

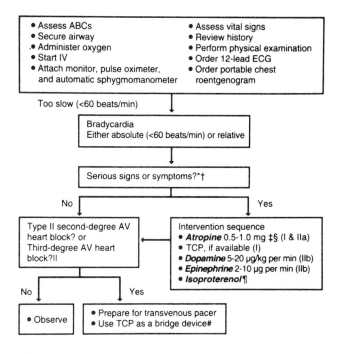

Assess ABCs	Assess vital signs
Secure airway	Review history
Administer oxygen	Perform physical examination
Start IV	Order 12-lead ECG
Attach monitor, pulse oximeter, and automatic sphygmomanometer	Order portable chest roentgenogram

Too slow (<60 beats/min)

Bradycardia
Either absolute (<60 beats/min) or relative

Serious signs or symptoms?*†

No | Yes

Type II second-degree AV heart block? or Third-degree AV heart block?‖

Intervention sequence
- *Atropine* 0.5-1.0 mg ‡§ (I & IIa)
- TCP, if available (I)
- *Dopamine* 5-20 µg/kg per min (IIb)
- *Epinephrine* 2-10 µg per min (IIb)
- *Isoproterenol*¶

No | Yes

- Observe

- Prepare for transvenous pacer
- Use TCP as a bridge device#

*Serious signs or symptoms must be related to the slow rate.
 Clinical manifestations include:
 symptoms (chest pain, shortness of breath, decreased level of consciousness) and
 signs (low BP, shock, pulmonary congestion, CHF, acute MI).
†Do not delay TCP while awaiting IV access or for *atropine* to take effect if patient is symptomatic.
‡Denervated transplanted hearts will not respond to *atropine*. Go at once to pacing, *catecholamine* infusion, or both.
§*Atropine* should be given in repeat doses in 3-5 min up to total of 0.04 mg/kg. Consider shorter dosing intervals in severe clinical conditions. It has been suggested that atropine should be used with caution in atrioventricular (AV) block at the His-Purkinje level (type II AV block and new third-degree block with wide QRS complexes) (Class IIb).
‖Never treat third-degree heart block plus ventricular escape beats with *lidocaine*.
¶*Isoproterenol* should be used, if at all, with exteme caution. At low doses it is Class IIb (possibly helpful); at higher doses it is Class III (harmful).
#Verify patient tolerance and mechanical capture. Use analgesia and sedation as needed.

Figure 5. Bradycardia algorithm.   *273*

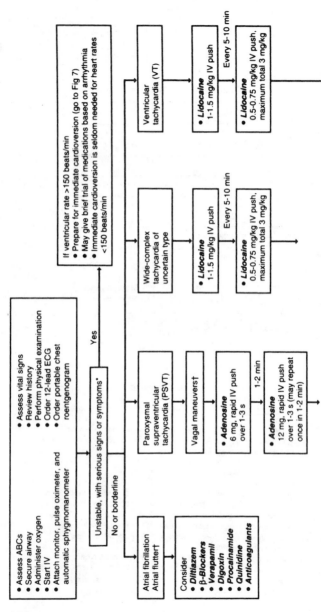

- Assess ABCs
- Secure airway
- Administer oxygen
- Start IV
- Attach monitor, pulse oximeter, and automatic sphygmomanometer
- Assess vital signs
- Review history
- Perform physical examination
- Order 12-lead ECG
- Order portable chest roentgenogram

Unstable, with serious signs or symptoms*

No or borderline

Yes

If ventricular rate >150 beats/min
- Prepare for immediate cardioversion (go to Fig 7)
- May give brief trial of medications based on arrhythmia
- Immediate cardioversion is seldom needed for heart rates <150 beats/min

Atrial fibrillation Atrial flutter

Consider
- *Diltiazem*
- *β-Blockers*
- *Verapamil*
- *Digoxin*
- *Procainamide*
- *Quinidine*
- *Anticoagulants*

Paroxysmal supraventricular tachycardia (PSVT)

Vagal maneuvers†

- *Adenosine* 6 mg, rapid IV push over 1-3 s

1-2 min

- *Adenosine* 12 mg, rapid IV push over 1-3 s (may repeat once in 1-2 min)

Wide-complex tachycardia of uncertain type

- *Lidocaine* 1-1.5 mg/kg IV push

Every 5-10 min

- *Lidocaine* 0.5-0.75 mg/kg IV push, maximum total 3 mg/kg

Ventricular tachycardia (VT)

- *Lidocaine* 1-1.5 mg/kg IV push

Every 5-10 min

- *Lidocaine* 0.5-0.75 mg/kg IV push, maximum total 3 mg/kg

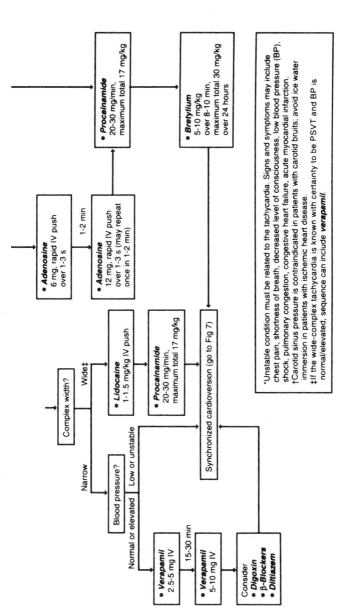

Figure 6. Tachycardia algorithm.

275

NOTES

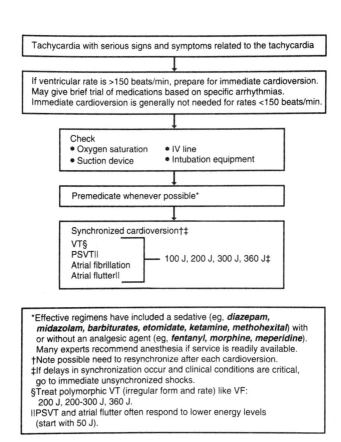

Tachycardia with serious signs and symptoms related to the tachycardia

If ventricular rate is >150 beats/min, prepare for immediate cardioversion.
May give brief trial of medications based on specific arrhythmias.
Immediate cardioversion is generally not needed for rates <150 beats/min.

Check
- Oxygen saturation
- Suction device
- IV line
- Intubation equipment

Premedicate whenever possible*

Synchronized cardioversion†‡
VT§
PSVT‖
Atrial fibrillation
Atrial flutter‖
— 100 J, 200 J, 300 J, 360 J‡

*Effective regimens have included a sedative (eg, *diazepam, midazolam, barbiturates, etomidate, ketamine, methohexital*) with or without an analgesic agent (eg, *fentanyl, morphine, meperidine*). Many experts recommend anesthesia if service is readily available.
†Note possible need to resynchronize after each cardioversion.
‡If delays in synchronization occur and clinical conditions are critical, go to immediate unsynchronized shocks.
§Treat polymorphic VT (irregular form and rate) like VF: 200 J, 200-300 J, 360 J.
‖PSVT and atrial flutter often respond to lower energy levels (start with 50 J).

Figure 7. Electrical cardioversion algorithm (with the patient not in cardiac arrest).

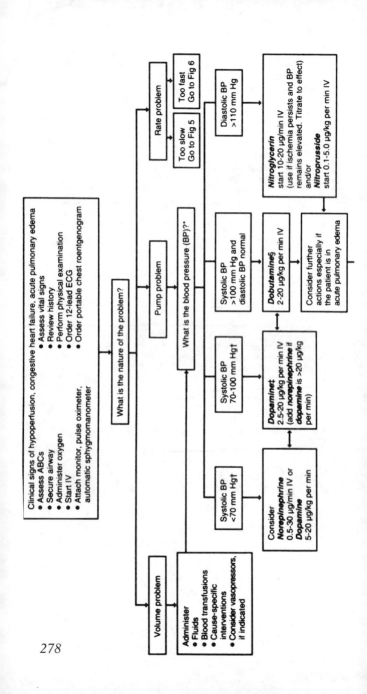

Clinical signs of hypoperfusion, congestive heart failure, acute pulmonary edema
• Assess ABCs   • Assess vital signs
• Secure airway   • Review history
• Administer oxygen   • Perform physical examination
• Start IV   • Order 12-lead ECG
• Attach monitor, pulse oximeter,   • Order portable chest roentgenogram
  automatic sphygmomanometer

What is the nature of the problem?

| Volume problem | Pump problem | Rate problem |

Volume problem

Administer
• Fluids
• Blood transfusions
• Cause-specific interventions
• Consider vasopressors, if indicated

Pump problem

What is the blood pressure (BP)?*

| Systolic BP <70 mm Hg† | Systolic BP 70-100 mm Hg† | Systolic BP >100 mm Hg and diastolic BP normal |

Consider
Norepinephrine
0.5-30 μg/min IV or
Dopamine
5-20 μg/kg per min

Dopamine‡
2.5-20 μg/kg per min IV
(add **norepinephrine** if
dopamine is >20 μg/kg
per min)

Dobutamine§
2-20 μg/kg per min IV

Consider further
actions especially if
the patient is in
acute pulmonary edema

Rate problem

| Too slow Go to Fig 5 | Too fast Go to Fig 6 |

Diastolic BP
>110 mm Hg

Nitroglycerin
start 10-20 μg/min IV
(use if ischemia persists and BP
remains elevated. Titrate to effect)
and/or
Nitroprusside
start 0.1-5.0 μg/kg per min IV

278

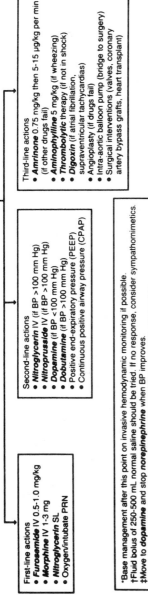

First-line actions
- **Furosemide** IV 0.5–1.0 mg/kg
- **Morphine** IV 1–3 mg
- **Nitroglycerin** SL
- Oxygen/intubate PRN

Second-line actions
- **Nitroglycerin** IV (if BP >100 mm Hg)
- **Nitroprusside** IV (if BP >100 mm Hg)
- **Dopamine** (if BP <100 mm Hg)
- **Dobutamine** (if BP >100 mm Hg)
- Positive end-expiratory pressure (PEEP)
- Continuous positive airway pressure (CPAP)

Third-line actions
- **Amrinone** 0.75 mg/kg then 5–15 µg/kg per min (if other drugs fail)
- **Aminophylline** 5 mg/kg (if wheezing)
- **Thrombolytic** therapy (if not in shock)
- **Digoxin** (if atrial fibrillation, supraventricular tachycardias)
- Angioplasty (if drugs fail)
- Intra-aortic balloon pump (bridge to surgery)
- Surgical interventions (valves, coronary artery bypass grafts, heart transplant)

*Base management after this point on invasive hemodynamic monitoring if possible.
†Fluid bolus of 250–500 mL normal saline should be tried. If no response, consider sympathomimetics.
‡Move to **dopamine** and stop **norepinephrine** when BP improves.
§Add **dopamine** (and avoid **dobutamine**) if systolic BP drops below 100 mm Hg.

Figure 8. Acute pulmonary edema/hypotension/shock algorithm.

279

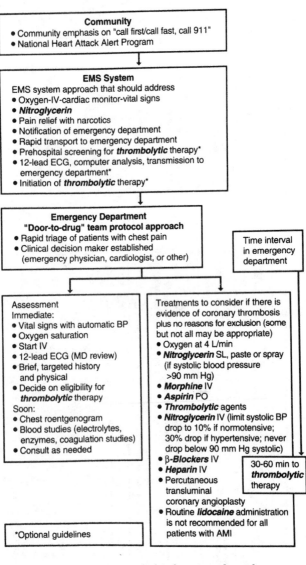

Community
- Community emphasis on "call first/call fast, call 911"
- National Heart Attack Alert Program

EMS System
EMS system approach that should address
- Oxygen-IV-cardiac monitor-vital signs
- *Nitroglycerin*
- Pain relief with narcotics
- Notification of emergency department
- Rapid transport to emergency department
- Prehospital screening for *thrombolytic* therapy*
- 12-lead ECG, computer analysis, transmission to emergency department*
- Initiation of *thrombolytic* therapy*

Emergency Department
"Door-to-drug" team protocol approach
- Rapid triage of patients with chest pain
- Clinical decision maker established (emergency physician, cardiologist, or other)

Time interval in emergency department

Assessment
Immediate:
- Vital signs with automatic BP
- Oxygen saturation
- Start IV
- 12-lead ECG (MD review)
- Brief, targeted history and physical
- Decide on eligibility for *thrombolytic* therapy
Soon:
- Chest roentgenogram
- Blood studies (electrolytes, enzymes, coagulation studies)
- Consult as needed

Treatments to consider if there is evidence of coronary thrombosis plus no reasons for exclusion (some but not all may be appropriate)
- Oxygen at 4 L/min
- *Nitroglycerin* SL, paste or spray (if systolic blood pressure >90 mm Hg)
- *Morphine* IV
- *Aspirin* PO
- *Thrombolytic* agents
- *Nitroglycerin* IV (limit systolic BP drop to 10% if normotensive; 30% drop if hypertensive; never drop below 90 mm Hg systolic)
- β-*Blockers* IV
- *Heparin* IV
- Percutaneous transluminal coronary angioplasty
- Routine *lidocaine* administration is not recommended for all patients with AMI

30-60 min to *thrombolytic* therapy

*Optional guidelines

Figure 9. Acute myocardial infarction algorithm.

280

Appendix B: Effects of Specific Toxins on Various Organ Systems

VITAL SIGNS

Tachycardia: Ethanol, sympathomimetics, anticholinergics, theophylline, withdrawal states, salicylates, thyroid supplements, lithium, monoamine oxidase (MAO) inhibitors, digoxin, ergot alkaloids, TCAs, neuroleptics, mushrooms, nicotine

Bradycardia: Beta-blockers, calcium-channel blockers, barbiturates, cholinergics, sedatives and hypnotics, digitalis, opioids, CO, cyanide, cimetidine, clonidine, lead, organophosphates, quinine

Tachypnea: Anticholinergics, amphetamines, hydrocarbons, metabolic acidosis (**MUDPILES**), CO, salicylates, organophosphates, theophylline, withdrawal states, camphor, clonidine, cocaine, ethanol, methanol, ethylene glycol, hydrocarbons

Bradypnea: Alcohols, barbiturates, opioids, sedatives and hypnotics, clonidine, CO, cyanide (late exposure)

Hypertension: Anticholinergics, sympathomimetics, amphetamines, thyroid supplements, withdrawal states, barium, cadmium, CO, clonidine withdrawal, corticosteroids, ergot alkaloids, lead, mercury, MAO inhibitors, nicotine, theophylline

Hypotension: Antihypertensives, sedatives, opioids, TCAs, iron, CO, cyanide, digitalis, nitrites, nitrates, mushrooms, barbiturates, disulfiram (Antabuse), procainamide, insecticides, LSD

Hyperthermia: Anticholinergics, sympathomimetics, phenothiazines, salicylates, TCAs, ethanol withdrawal, amphetamines, betablockers, atropine, iron, antihistamines, herbicides, metal fumes, thyroid supplements, theophylline, snake venom

Hypothermia: Barbiturates, opioids, sedatives, TCAs, alcohol, hypoglycemic agents, CO, cyanide, ethanol, clonidine, antipsychotics, hydrogen sulfide

NEUROLOGIC EXAMINATION

Miosis (pinpoint pupils): Use the mnemonic **POOPP: P** = PCP; **O** = opioids (except meperidine, diphenoxylate, dextromethorphan); **O** = organophosphates and cholinergics; **P** = phenothiazines; **P** = pontine hemorrhage. Also barbiturates (late) and nicotine

Mydriasis (dilated pupils): Use the mnemonic **SAW: S** = sympathomimetics; **A** = anticholinergics; **W** = withdrawal of substances of abuse. Also phenytoin, glutethimide, barbiturates, xanthines, cimetidine, and antihistamines

Seizures: Use the mnemonic **CAP: C** = carbon monoxide, camphor, cocaine, cyanide, chlorinated hydrocarbons; **A** = anticholinergics, aspirin, amphetamines/sympathomimetics, aminophylline, alcohols, ammonia, arsenic; **P** = PCP, phenothiazines, pesticides, phenytoin, propoxyphene, phenol. Also lead, lithium, carbamazepine, strychnine, antidepressants, and hypoglycemic agents

Nystagmus: Phenytoin, carbamazepine, barbiturates, glutethimide, salicylates, CO, alcohols, sedatives, PCP (often rotatory)

Toxic psychosis: Sympathomimetics, anticholinergics, hallucinogens, heavy metals, carbon disulfide

Violent behavior: PCP, cocaine, amphetamines, ethanol

THE SKIN

Cyanosis: Nitrates, nitrites, sulfonamides, aniline dyes

Dry, flushed skin: Anticholinergics, botulinum toxin

Profuse sweating: Cholinergics, anticholinesterases, sympathomimetics, salicylates, ethanol withdrawal, dinitrophenol

Bullae: Barbiturates, CO, ethchlorvynol, hexachlorbenzene, scombroid poisoning

Skin discoloration: *Blue:* oxalic acid; *bronze:* arsine; *brown:* bromides, iodine, nitrates, nitrites, phenytoin, local anesthetics; *gray-black:* chloramphenicol, silver; *orange:* nitric acid; *red:* antihistamines, anticholinergics, CO, cyanide, boric acid, rifampin, vancomycin, mercury; *yellow:* carotenoids, epoxy resins, rifampin

Needle tracks: Opioids, cocaine

Purpura: Anticoagulants, quinine, salicylates, snake and spider bites

Piloerection: Withdrawal states

DIAGNOSTIC ODORS

Acetone: Lacquer, alcohol, ketoacidosis, chloroform, isopropyl alcohol, phenol, salicylates

Bitter almonds: cyanide, silver polish

Stove gas: CO (odorless yet associated with stove gas)

Fruit-like: Amyl nitrite, chloral hydrate, ethanol

Rotten eggs: Hydrogen sulfide, disulfiram (Antabuse), mercaptens

Wintergreen: Methyl salicylate

Moth balls: Naphthalene, camphor

Shoe polish: Nitrobenzenes

Ammonia: Uremia

Garlic: Arsenic, organophosphates, selenium, malathion, parathion, thallium, dimethylsulfoxide

Index

An "f" following a page number indicates a figure; a "t" indicates a table.